Urodynamics

Editors

BENJAMIN M. BRUCKER
VICTOR W. NITTI

UROLOGIC CLINICS
OF NORTH AMERICA

www.urologic.theclinics.com

Consulting Editor
SAMIR S. TANEJA

August 2014 • Volume 41 • Number 3

ELSEVIER

1600 John F. Kennedy Boulevard • Suite 1800 • Philadelphia, Pennsylvania, 19103-2899

http://www.theclinics.com

UROLOGIC CLINICS OF NORTH AMERICA Volume 41, Number 3
August 2014 ISSN 0094-0143, ISBN-13: 978-0-323-32027-6

Editor: Kerry Holland
Developmental Editor: Susan Showalter

Urologic Clinics of North America (ISSN 0094-0143) is published quarterly by Elsevier Inc., 360 Park Avenue South, New York, NY 10010-1710. Months of issue are February, May, August, and November. Business and Editorial Offices: 1600 John F. Kennedy Blvd., Suite 1800, Philadelphia, PA 19103-2899. Periodicals postage paid at New York, NY and additional mailing offices. Subscription prices are $355.00 per year (US individuals), $602.00 per year (US institutions), $415.00 per year (Canadian individuals), $752.00 per year (Canadian institutions), $515.00 per year (foreign individuals), and $752.00 per year (foreign institutions). Foreign air speed delivery is included in all *Clinics* subscription prices. All prices are subject to change without notice. **POSTMASTER:** Send address changes to *Urologic Clinics of North America*, Elsevier Health Sciences Division, Subscription Customer Service, 3251 Riverport Lane, Maryland Heights, MO 63043. Customer Service: 1-800-654-2452 (US). From outside the United States, call 1-314-447-8871. Fax: 1-314-447-8029. E-mail: JournalsCustomerServiceusa@elsevier.com (for print support) and JournalsOnlineSupport-usa@elsevier.com (for online support).

Reprints. For copies of 100 or more, of articles in this publication, please contact the Commercial Reprints Department, Elsevier Inc., 360 Park Avenue South, New York, New York 10010-1710. Tel.: 212-633-3874; Fax: 212-633-3820; E-mail: reprints@elsevier.com.

Urologic Clinics of North America is covered in MEDLINE/PubMed (*Index Medicus*), *Excerpta Medica, Current Contents/ Clinical Medicine, Science Citation Index,* and *ISI/BIOMED*.

PROGRAM OBJECTIVE
The goal of *Urologic Clinics of North America* is to keep practicing urologists and urology residents up to date with current clinical practice in urology by providing timely articles reviewing the state of the art in patient care.

TARGET AUDIENCE
Practicing urologists, urology residents and other health care professionals practicing in the discipline of urology.

LEARNING OBJECTIVES
Upon completion of this activity, participants will be able to:
1. Review the American Urologic Association/Society of Urodynamics, Female Pelvic Medicine and Urogential Reconstruction (SUFU) adult urodynamics guideline.
2. Discuss the necessity and use of urodynamics in stress incontinence.
3. Recognize the keys to good practice in urodynamic study.

ACCREDITATION
The Elsevier Office of Continuing Medical Education (EOCME) is accredited by the Accreditation Council for Continuing Medical Education (ACCME) to provide continuing medical education for physicians.

The EOCME designates this enduring material for a maximum of 15 *AMA PRA Category 1 Credit*(s)™. Physicians should claim only the credit commensurate with the extent of their participation in the activity.

All other health care professionals requesting continuing education credit for this enduring material will be issued a certificate of participation.

DISCLOSURE OF CONFLICTS OF INTEREST
The EOCME assesses conflict of interest with its instructors, faculty, planners, and other individuals who are in a position to control the content of CME activities. All relevant conflicts of interest that are identified are thoroughly vetted by EOCME for fair balance, scientific objectivity, and patient care recommendations. EOCME is committed to providing its learners with CME activities that promote improvements or quality in healthcare and not a specific proprietary business or a commercial interest.

The planning committee, staff, authors and editors listed below have identified no financial relationships or relationships to products or devices they or their spouse/life partner have with commercial interest related to the content of this CME activity:
Katie N. Ballert, MD; Benjamin Brucker, MD; Lysanne Campeau, MD, PhD, FRCSC; Clinton W. Collins, MD; Lindsey Cox, MD; Teresa L. Danforth, MD; Benjamin E. Dillon, MD; David A. Ginsberg, MD; Howard B. Goldman, MD, FACS; Kerry Holland; Brynne Hunter; William I. Jaffe, MD; Ying Hua Jura, MD; Indu Kumari; Sandy Lavery; Gary Lemack, MD; Lara MacLachlan, MD; Brian K. Marks, MD; Jill McNair; Sylvester Onyishi, MD; Lindsay Parnell; Lisa M. Parrillo, MD; Parvati Ramchandani, MD; Eric S. Rovner, MD; Harriette Scarpero, MD; Ariana Smith, MD.

The planning committee, staff, authors and editors listed below have identified financial relationships or relationships to products or devices they or their spouse/life partner have with commercial interest related to the content of this CME activity:
Craig V. Comiter, MD is a consultant/advisor for Coloplast.

Victor W. Nitti, MD is a consultant advisor for Allergan Inc., American Medical Systems Inc., Astellas Pharma US, Inc., Coloplast, Pfizer Inc., Pneumoflex Systems LLC, TheraCoat and Serenity Pharmaceuticals Corp.; is on speakers bureau for Allergan Inc., and has stock ownership with Serenity Pharmaceuticals Corp.

Samir S. Taneja, MD; is a consultant/advisor for Eigen Pharma LLC, GTx, Inc., Bayer Healthcare Pharmaceuticals, Healthtronics, Inc. and Hitachi, Ltd.

Christian Twiss, MD; is on speakers bureau for Astellas Pharma US, Inc.

J. Christian Winters, MD is a consultant/advisor for Pfizer Inc., Allergan Inc, Astellas Pharma US, Inc. and Solace Pharmaceuticals Inc.

UNAPPROVED/OFF-LABEL USE DISCLOSURE
The EOCME requires CME faculty to disclose to the participants:
1. When products or procedures being discussed are off-label, unlabelled, experimental, and/or investigational (not US Food and Drug Administration (FDA) approved); and
2. Any limitations on the information presented, such as data that are preliminary or that represent ongoing research, interim analyses, and/or unsupported opinions. Faculty may discuss information about pharmaceutical agents that is outside of FDA-approved labelling. This information is intended solely for CME and is not intended to promote off-label use of these medications. If you have any questions, contact the medical affairs department of the manufacturer for the most recent prescribing information.

TO ENROLL
To enroll in the *Urologic Clinics of North America* Continuing Medical Education program, call customer service at 1-800-654-2452 or sign up online at http://www.theclinics.com/home/cme. The CME program is available to subscribers for an additional annual fee of $270 USD.

METHOD OF PARTICIPATION

In order to claim credit, participants must complete the following:

1. Complete enrolment as indicated above.
2. Read the activity.
3. Complete the CME Test and Evaluation. Participants must achieve a score of 70% on the test. All CME Tests and Evaluations must be completed online.

CME INQUIRIES/SPECIAL NEEDS

For all CME inquiries or special needs, please contact elsevierCME@elsevier.com.

Contributors

CONSULTING EDITOR

SAMIR S. TANEJA, MD
The James M. Neissa and Janet Riha Neissa
Professor of Urologic Oncology; Professor of
Urology and Radiology; Director, Division of
Urologic Oncology, Department of Urology;
Co-Director, Smilow Comprehensive Prostate
Cancer Center, New York University Langone
Medical Center, New York, New York

EDITORS

BENJAMIN M. BRUCKER, MD
Assistant Professor, Department of Urology;
Director of Neurourology, MS Comprehensive
Care Center, New York University Langone
Medical Center, New York, New York

VICTOR W. NITTI, MD
Professor of Urology and Obstetrics and
Gynecology; Vice-Chairman, Department of
Urology, New York University Langone Medical
Center, New York, New York

AUTHORS

KATIE N. BALLERT, MD
Assistant Professor, Division of Urology,
Department of Surgery, University of Kentucky,
Lexington, Kentucky

LYSANNE CAMPEAU, MD, PhD, FRCSC
Assistant Professor, Division of Urology,
Department of Surgery, Jewish General
Hospital, Lady Davis Institute for Medical
Research, McGill University, Montreal,
Quebec, Canada

CLINTON W. COLLINS, MD
Assistant Professor, Division of Urology,
University of Mississippi Health Sciences
Center, Jackson, Mississippi

CRAIG V. COMITER, MD
Department of Urology, Stanford University
School of Medicine, Stanford, California

LINDSEY COX, MD
Fellow, Female Pelvic Medicine and
Reconstructive Surgery, Department of
Urology, University of Michigan, Ann Arbor,
Michigan

TERESA L. DANFORTH, MD
Assistant Professor and Associate Program
Director, Department of Urology, SUNY Buffalo
School of Medicine and Biomedical Sciences,
Buffalo General Hospital, Buffalo, New York

BENJAMIN E. DILLON, MD
Department of Urology, Kelsey-Seybold Clinic,
Houston, Texas

DAVID A. GINSBERG, MD
Associate Professor, Department of Urology,
Keck School of Medicine of USC, University
of Southern California, Los Angeles, California

HOWARD B. GOLDMAN, MD
Professor, Lerner College of Medicine,
Glickman Urological and Kidney Institute,
Cleveland Clinic, Cleveland, Ohio

WILLIAM I. JAFFE, MD
Assistant Professor of Urology, Division of
Urology, Department of Surgery, Perelman
Center for Advanced Medicine, University
of Pennsylvania, Philadelphia, Pennsylvania

YING H. JURA, MD
Department of Urology, Stanford University
School of Medicine, Stanford, California

GARY E. LEMACK, MD
Professor of Urology and Neurology,
Department of Urology, University of Texas
Southwestern Medical Center, Dallas, Texas

LARA S. MACLACHLAN, MD
Department of Urology, Medical University
of South Carolina, Charleston, South Carolina

BRIAN K. MARKS, MD
Center for Urologic Care, Concord Hospital,
Concord, New Hampshire

SYLVESTER E. ONYISHI, MD
Urology Resident, Division of Urology,
University of Arizona College of Medicine,
Tucson, Arizona

LISA M. PARRILLO, MD
Resident in Urology, Division of Urology,
Department of Surgery, Hospital of the
University of Pennsylvania, Philadelphia,
Pennsylvania

PARVATI RAMCHANDANI, MD
Professor of Radiology and Surgery, Division
of Urology, Department of Surgery, Hospital of
the University of Pennsylvania; Department
of Radiology, Hospital of the University of
Pennsylvania, Philadelphia, Pennsylvania

ERIC S. ROVNER, MD
Professor, Department of Urology, Medical
University of South Carolina, Charleston,
South Carolina

HARRIETTE SCARPERO, MD
Associated Urologists, Nashville, Tennessee

ARIANA L. SMITH, MD
Assistant Professor of Urology in Surgery,
Division of Urology, Department of Surgery,
Perelman School of Medicine, Philadelphia,
Pennsylvania

CHRISTIAN O. TWISS, MD, FACS
Director of Female Urology, Pelvic Medicine,
and Pelvic Reconstructive Surgery; Associate
Professor of Surgery, Division of Urology,
University of Arizona College of Medicine,
Tucson, Arizona

J. CHRISTIAN WINTERS, MD, FACS
H. Eustis Reily Professor and Chairman,
Department of Urology, Louisiana State
University Health Sciences Center,
New Orleans, Louisiana

Contents

specialized study as well as technique. Appropriate and judicious use of fluoro-urodynamics lends to improved diagnostic acumen in a well-selected patient population; however, clinicians must be mindful of the added cost, safety concerns, and limitations of its use.

Stress urinary incontinence is a prevalent condition that significantly impairs the quality of life. This article presents a critical summary of the current literature on the use and value of urodynamic studies in the evaluation of stress urinary incontinence in women.

In this article, the value of urodynamic studies in the evaluation of treatment of male lower urinary tract symptoms is appraised based on current evidence. The information gained by urodynamics can be a valuable tool for counseling patients considering invasive outlet reduction procedures.

The routine use of preoperative urodynamics in the woman considering surgery for pelvic organ prolapse is a topic of much debate. This article addresses the use of urodynamics in patients with pelvic organ prolapse. It specifically discusses the utility of urodynamics in the evaluation stress incontinence on prolapse reduction (occult stress urinary incontinence) as well as concomitant storage and voiding symptoms in these patients.

Urodynamics is indicated for the evaluation of postprostatectomy incontinence unless an artificial urinary sphincter placement is the preferred option, as in cases of severe incontinence, prior radiation, or previous male sling or artificial urinary sphincter placement—when male sling is unlikely to achieve efficacy. Urodynamics should be performed only when there is a question it can answer that would affect treatment choice or outcome. Urodynamic findings of detrusor underactivity, overactivity, and reduced compliance are important considerations in deciding how best to treat postprostatectomy incontinence.

Urodynamics remains the test of choice to evaluate lower urinary tract symptoms in men and women. Best practices recommend that urodynamics be applied to answer a specific urodynamic question. Recent level 1 evidence shows that urodynamics is not necessary for the evaluation of pure clinical stress urinary incontinence. Urodynamics is also not needed before conservative treatment of overactive bladder. Urodynamics still has an important role in the evaluation of mixed urinary incontinence and voiding lower urinary tract symptoms. The information obtained assists the clinician in confirmation of the diagnosis, counseling the patient, and choosing treatment.

Multiple sclerosis (MS) is an autoimmune inflammatory disease that results in damage to the myelin sheaths of the nerves in the central nervous system. Urinary urgency, frequency, and urgency incontinence are the most common symptoms, occurring in 37% to 99% of patients. Voiding symptoms (hesitancy, feeling of incomplete bladder emptying, and occasionally urinary retention) are also common in this population, occurring in 34% to 79% of patients. Traditionally, filling cystometry combined with pressure/flow studies has been a cornerstone of the initial evaluation of all patients with neurogenic lower urinary tract dysfunction, although recently that practice has been challenged.

Neurogenic lower urinary tract dysfunction (NLUTD) affects many patients and requires close monitoring. Initial studies establishing patients at risk for upper tract disease revealed that high detrusor leak point pressures were predictive of upper tract disease. Urodynamics in patients with NLUTD have specific challenges. Initial studies in patients after an acute injury should be delayed until after the spinal shock phase. In children with spinal dysraphism, studies should be done early to established potential risk. The goals are maintaining low bladder pressures, decreasing risk of infection, and maintaining continence.

There are well established pressure flow criteria and nomograms for urinary obstruction in men. The pressure flow criteria for female urinary obstruction are not well established due to differences in female voiding dynamics as compared to men. Typically, other information such as radiographic data and clinical symptoms are needed to facilitate the diagnosis. Detrusor underactivity remains a poorly studied clinical condition without definitive urodynamic diagnostic criteria. Modalities proposed for objective analysis of detrusor function such as power (watt) factor, linear passive urethral resistance relation and BCI nomogram were all developed to analyze male voiding dysfunction. Overall, further investigation is needed to establish acceptable urodynamic criteria for defining detrusor underactivity in women.

UROLOGIC CLINICS OF NORTH AMERICA

Foreword
Urodynamics

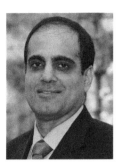

Samir S. Taneja, MD
Consulting Editor

The management of the voiding dysfunction has evolved greatly over the past 20 years from an approach of therapeutic trial and error to an approach of selective data gathering and individually formulated therapeutic strategies. The core of this more informed approach is urodynamic testing. The test provides data regarding the nature of voiding dysfunction, and, in doing so, provides a basis for individualized pharmacologic and surgical strategies.

One could argue that the tremendous advances in the pharmacologic management of bladder dysfunction have been made possible by the data provided through urodynamic testing. By providing a metric for assessing therapeutic response, efficacy could be better assessed and titrated. In a similar manner, surgical therapy has been refined in patients with obstructive urinary dysfunction and in those with incontinence. Urodynamics have not only provided a measure of success for therapy, but, more importantly, the testing has allowed strict indications for surgical intervention to be defined.

The use of urodynamics in clinical practice has gone from a rarely used tool to one that is, perhaps, overutilized due to wide availability and financial incentive. The testing has clear indications, and its use should be among those patients in whom management would clearly be influenced by outcome. Instructing urologists in the clear indications for and practice of urodynamics will be a necessary challenge for our field in the emerging era of health care reform. As such, this issue of *Urologic Clinics of North America* devoted to urodynamics is extremely timely.

The practice of urodynamics is constantly evolving. In this issue, I have asked my colleagues, Drs Benjamin Brucker and Victor Nitti, to provide us with an update of urodynamic testing, including indications, interpretation, and the impact of outcome on clinical management in common disorders. In doing so, they commissioned a comprehensive group of articles from our field's leading experts, encompassing many of the common scenarios in which urologists are asked to assess voiding dysfunction. I am deeply indebted to Drs Brucker and Nitti, and the authors of these articles, who have provided a wonderful perspective on clinical management. Given the considerable impact of voiding dysfunction on the average urology practice, I have no doubt the articles will serve as a valuable resource for our readers.

Samir S. Taneja, MD
Division of Urologic Oncology
Smilow Comprehensive Prostate Cancer Center
Department of Urology
NYU Langone Medical Center
150 East 32nd Street, Suite 200
New York, NY 10016, USA

E-mail address:
samir.taneja@nyumc.org

Urol Clin N Am 41 (2014) xi
http://dx.doi.org/10.1016/j.ucl.2014.07.001
0094-0143/14/$ – see front matter © 2014 Published by Elsevier Inc.

urologic.theclinics.com

Preface
Urodynamics

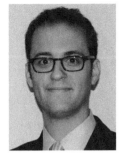 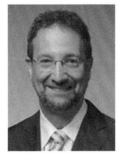

Benjamin M. Brucker, MD   Victor W. Nitti, MD

Editors

Lower urinary tract dysfunction and its associated symptoms can be a significant burden to those who are affected. Whether it be lower urinary tract symptoms or upper tract consequences, there can be a tremendous negative impact of health-related quality of life in both men and women. Urodynamics, by studying how the lower urinary tract stores and empties, can be a critical tool in the management of patients, but should not be used indiscriminately. In the evaluation of patients with lower urinary tract dysfunction and lower urinary tract symptoms, clinicians should ask two critical questions: When are urodynamics helpful? and how will the information obtained influence patient management?

Although these two questions are straightforward, the answers can be extremely complex. This complexity can cause confusion in many people's minds about the role of urodynamics in clinical practice. The urodynamic study must be done in an appropriately selected situation with a specific question in mind; it must be a well-executed high-quality study, and the results must be interpreted carefully in the appropriate clinical context.

As guest editors for this issue of *Urologic Clinics of North America*, it was our goal to provide readers with some of the tools that they will need to understand the subtle nuances of this field. The issue starts with the most up-to-date guidelines and practices and then takes the reader through some of the most common conditions that may require urodynamic investigation. After reading this issue cover to cover (or savoring each gem of an article), we have no doubt it will find a home on the office shelf next to the urodynamic unit user manual and be referenced often. It will help teach the less experienced urodynamicist and will update the more experienced with the latest clinical evidence. There are situations where urodynamics can have tremendous value, and these are highlighted in the following pages. But, just as importantly, there are limitations and shortcomings of these interactive studies that are also appropriately acknowledged.

The authors of these of articles include some of the brightest stars in our field. You will quickly understand, as you read their work, why we hand-selected each and every author. We are grateful that they agreed to work with us to provide this critically important review of urodynamics.

Benjamin M. Brucker, MD
Department of Urology
New York University Langone Medical Center
150 East 32nd Street, Second Floor
New York, NY 10016, USA

Victor W. Nitti, MD
Department of Urology
New York University Langone Medical Center
150 East 32nd Street, Second Floor
New York, NY 10016, USA

E-mail addresses:
Benjamin.brucker@nyumc.org (B.M. Brucker)
Victor.Nitti@nyumc.org (V.W. Nitti)

Urol Clin N Am 41 (2014) xiii
http://dx.doi.org/10.1016/j.ucl.2014.06.001
0094-0143/14/$ – see front matter © 2014 Elsevier Inc. All rights reserved.

AUA/SUFU Adult Urodynamics Guideline
A Clinical Review

 CrossMark

Clinton W. Collins, MD[a], J. Christian Winters, MD[b],*

KEYWORDS

- Uroflow • PVR • Pressure-flow study • Videourodymanics • Cystometrogram • Overactive bladder
- Stress urinary incontinence • Lower urinary tract symptoms • Pelvic organ prolapse
- Neurogenic bladder

KEY POINTS

- In women with stress urinary incontinence (SUI), urodynamics (UDS) is an option in the preoperative assessment.
- If UDS is performed, urethral function should be measured.
- In patients with urinary urgency incontinence and mixed incontinence, the absence of detrusor overactivity (DO) on a single urodynamic study does not exclude it as a causative agent for their symptoms.
- Patients with relevant neurogenic conditions (at risk for upper tract complications) should undergo multichannel cystometrogram or pressure flow study (PFS) whether they have symptoms or not.
- The only way to accurately diagnose bladder outlet obstruction (BOO) is by PFS.

INTRODUCTION

UDS has long been considered a useful tool for the diagnosis and treatment of lower urinary tract symptoms (LUTS), incontinence, voiding dysfunction, and neurogenic bladder. There has been recent controversy regarding the specific role of UDS. The Value of Urodynamic Education (ValUE) trial reported no improvement in 12-month outcomes between women with stress-predominant urinary incontinence randomized preoperatively to an office evaluation alone versus office evaluation plus preoperative UDS. However, diagnoses were changed in some patients who underwent UDS, as the surgeons were more likely to diagnose intrinsic sphincteric deficiency and less likely to diagnose overactive bladder (OAB), suggesting that UDS did change the clinician's diagnosis before surgery.[1] The utility of pressure-flow studies (PFS) in men before surgery for LUTS secondary to benign prostatic enlargement has long been debated.[2,3] The American Urological Association (AUA) and the Society of Urodynamics Female Pelvic Medicine and Urogenital Reconstruction (SUFU) published guidelines for the use of UDS in adults, and this article reviews this update and places these findings in clinical perspective.

Traditionally, physicians have used UDS for the following scenarios: (1) to identify factors contributing to lower urinary tract dysfunction and assess their relevance, (2) to predict the consequences of lower urinary tract dysfunction on the upper tracts, (3) to predict the consequences and outcomes of therapeutic intervention, (4) to confirm and/or understand the effects of interventional techniques, and (5) to investigate the reasons for treatment failure.[4] Because pretesting anxiety and urethral catheterization is necessary for some forms of

[a] Division of Urology, University of Mississippi Health Sciences Center, 2500 North State Street, Jackson, MS 39216, USA; [b] Department of Urology, Louisiana State University Health Sciences Center, 1542 Tulane Avenue, Room 547, New Orleans, LA 70112, USA
* Corresponding author.
E-mail address: cwinte@lsuhsc.edu

Urol Clin N Am 41 (2014) 353–362
http://dx.doi.org/10.1016/j.ucl.2014.04.011
0094-0143/14/$ – see front matter © 2014 Elsevier Inc. All rights reserved.

UDS, the risks (bleeding, infection, urethral trauma, and pain) should be weighed with the potential benefits. UDS is not a static diagnostic examination that provides a diagnosis for lower urinary tract conditions. UDS is an interactive examination, which assesses lower urinary tract function and serves as an adjunct to the comprehensive evaluation of patients with LUTS. In most patients presenting with lower urinary tract disorders, UDS is usually not necessary in the routine initial evaluation or even before empiric treatment in most cases. The clinician should always formulate the urodynamic questions before any examination. The physician should always ask, "What am I hoping to gain from this test? What conditions do I need to assess during UDS testing? What symptoms need to be reproduced during the examination? And, will this test likely change my treatment plan?" If the physician cannot answer these questions and ensure that the patient complaints are reproduced, it is unlikely that the testing will be beneficial.[5]

The AUA/SUFU Urodynamics Guideline in adults reviewed publications from January 1990 through March 2011 with focus on the use of postvoid residual (PVR), uroflowmetry, cystometry, PFS, videourodynamic studies (VUDS), electromyography (EMG), and urethral function tests (Valsalva leak point pressure [VLPP], urethral pressure profile). These UDS tests were evaluated by themselves or if used in combination with any other UDS test. Four lower urinary tract conditions were assessed: stress incontinence and pelvic organ prolapse (POP), urinary urgency and urgency incontinence, LUTS (comprising predominately obstructive symptoms), and neurogenic bladder. The role of UDS in these urinary conditions was evaluated in 4 categories: diagnosis, prognosis, clinical management decisions, and patient outcomes. Studies that did not report findings separately for men and women were excluded. The AUA methodology for Guidelines Statements was used. Each guideline statement is based on the strength of the evidence and is standard in the AUA Guidelines process.[6,7] The nomenclature system for establishing guideline statement based on levels of evidence is included in **Table 1**.

These guidelines offer guidance statements with attention given to certain clinical scenarios, represented by the various lower urinary tract conditions within the guideline. The guideline statements represent the role of UDS in the evaluation in management of patients with these urinary disorders. Thus, the intent of this guideline is that following a symptom assessment, physical examination, and incontinence assessment, physicians can determine which scenario, and thus which recommendation, fits their patient. These differences in clinical presentation often guide the decision of whether UDS is indicated or not. Taking the guidelines into consideration, it is ultimately the physician's decision regarding what is best for each patient.

There are a total of 19 Guidelines Statements in each of the 4 clinical conditions. This article presents each Guideline Statement and offers clinical context and case scenarios.

STRESS URINARY INCONTINENCE AND PELVIC ORGAN PROLAPSE

1. Clinicians who are making the diagnosis of urodynamic stress incontinence should assess urethral function. (Recommendation; Evidence Strength: Grade C)

Table 1
AUA nomenclature system

Statement Type: Definition	Evidence Strength
Standards: Directive statements that an action should (benefits outweigh risks/burdens) or should not (risks/burdens outweigh benefits) be undertaken	Grade A or B
Recommendations: Directive statements that an action should (benefits outweigh risks/burdens) or should not (risks/burdens outweigh benefits) be undertaken	Grade C
Options: Nondirective because the balance between benefits and risks/burdens seems equal or unclear	Grade A, B, or C
Clinical Principle: Statement about a component of clinical care that is widely agreed upon by urologists or other clinicians	Insufficient publications to address certain questions from an evidence basis
Expert Opinion: Statement achieved by consensus of the Panel that is based on members' clinical training, experience, knowledge, and judgment	There may be no evidence

A. During multichannel UDS testing, all the instrumentation is in place to assess urethral function (without additional procedures). The assessment of urethral function is performed by the following tests:
   i. Urethral pressure profilometry/maximal urethral closure pressure
   ii. Abdominal leak point pressure (ALPP) (Valsalva/cough leak point pressure)— this measurement is easily obtained during demonstration of urodynamic SUI.
B. Because some treatments have been shown to be less effective in patients with poor urethral function,[8–10] it is recommended that urethral function be evaluated when UDS has been determined beneficial in the preoperative evaluation of SUI. In surgeons performing midurethral sling procedures, there are data suggesting that a retropubic sling is more effective in patients with intrinsic sphincteric deficiency.[11] Thus, there may be benefit in the assessment of urethral function in patients already selected for UDS before surgical intervention to help decide which procedure may be most effective.

2. Surgeons considering invasive therapy in patients with SUI should assess PVR urine volume. (Expert Opinion)
   A. Although the exact threshold for elevated PVR is not clearly defined, it seems prudent that before performing surgery for SUI, which will have an effect on outlet function, a PVR assessment should be performed to provide information on the emptying status before surgery. The PVR assessment is safe, of little risk, and serves as a screen for disorders of emptying that may be identified preoperatively. In addition, this value can be a useful comparison in patients who develop emptying symptoms after surgery.
   B. Usually, more than one PVR value should be obtained, and an elevated PVR should prompt further testing.

3. Clinicians may perform multichannel UDS in patients with both symptoms and physical findings of SUI who are considering invasive, potentially morbid, or irreversible treatments. (Option; Evidence Strength: Grade C)
   A. Information obtained from a UDS study before surgery can confirm the diagnosis and as stated earlier may facilitate selection of the surgical procedure. In addition, these studies may provide other confounding data (DO or impaired contractility) that may enhance preoperative counseling. Although it is routinely accepted as an option in the evaluation of an uncomplicated case of SUI, preoperative UDS can be considered to obtain additional information. Although studies have not shown improved outcomes with the addition of UDS to the preoperative evaluation, diagnoses and treatment decisions were altered in some cases.[1,12]
   B. In complex, complicated patients, preoperative UDS may be particularly helpful. These recommendations are congruent with the AUA Guidelines in the Surgical Management of SUI. That Guideline listed several indications for further UDS testing, including the inability to make a definitive diagnosis based on symptoms and initial evaluation; the presence of mixed incontinence; prior surgery to the urinary tract, including anti-incontinence procedures; known or suspected neurogenic bladder; negative stress test; elevated PVR; grade III or greater POP; and any evidence of dysfunctional voiding (**Table 2**).[13]

4. Clinicians should perform repeat stress testing with the urethral catheter removed in patients suspected of having SUI who do not demonstrate this finding with the catheter in place during UDS. (Recommendation; Evidence Strength: Grade C)
   A. Some patients who complain of SUI or demonstrate SUI on examination may not leak during UDS with the catheter in place. It is recommended that these women should have their urethral catheter removed and stress testing repeated without the catheter in place. More than 50% of women with SUI symptoms and up to 35% of men with post-prostatectomy incontinence who do not demonstrate SUI with the urethral catheter in place do so when it is removed.[14,15]
      i. In practice, the voiding study (PFS) is performed with the catheter in place, the bladder is filled with this catheter, and the catheter is removed for the attempt at demonstrating SUI with the catheter removed. Alternatively, the catheter is removed, SUI is demonstrated with the catheter out, and an uncontaminated catheter is replaced for completion of PFS.

5. In women with high-grade POP but without the symptom of SUI, clinicians should perform stress testing with reduction of the prolapse. Multichannel UDS with prolapse reduction may be used to assess for occult stress incontinence and detrusor dysfunction in these women with associated LUTS. (Option; Evidence Strength: Grade C)
   A. Patients with high-grade anterior and middle compartment prolapse should undergo

Table 2
Clinical case scenario 1 (SUI)

42-y-Old with Chief Complaint of SUI	42-y-Old with Chief Complaint of SUI

Symptoms:
  Leaks with exertion
  Denies difficulty emptying
  No urgency symptoms or UUI
	Symptoms:
	  Leaks with exertion
	  Denies difficulty emptying
	  Has moderate urgency without UUI

History:
  No prior GU surgery
  No comorbidity
	History:
	  Previous bladder lift
	  No comorbidity

Physical examination:
  Urethral hypermobility
  No prolapse
  + Stress test
  PVR 20 mL
	Physical examination:
	  Urethral hypermobility
	  No prolapse
	  + Stress test
	  PVR 20 mL

Recommendation:
  Discussion of treatment options
	Recommendation:
	  Pressure flow studies with ALPP assessment

Discussion:
  In this patient, the scenario is that of
  uncomplicated SUI symptoms with a normal
  PVR and positive stress test result. It is
  reasonable in this scenario to proceed to
  discussion of treatment options including
  surgery without UDS tests
	Discussion:
	  In this patient, the scenario is that of complex
	  storage symptoms of urgency and SUI. In
	  addition, a previous procedure was
	  performed. This scenario is more
	  complicated, and preoperative UDS may be
	  helpful. When doing UDS in this complex
	  setting, urethral function should be
	  measured

Abbreviations: GU, genitourinary; UUI, urgency urinary incontinence.

stress testing with the prolapse reduced. In these patients without LUTS, a stress test without the prolapse is all that may be needed, if the decision to repair the prolapse has been made. In women with concomitant LUTS, this may be performed during multichannel UDS testing to evaluate these symptoms.[16]

B. There are a significant number of women who have occult SUI (stress incontinence demonstrated after reduction of the prolapse) detected, and surgical intervention for SUI should be considered in these patients.[17,18]

C. Those performing prolapse reduction should be mindful that the instruments used to reduce prolapse (pessary, vaginal pack, or ring forceps) can produce BOO by compressing the urethra, which may mask SUI or increase VLPP (**Table 3**).

OVERACTIVE BLADDER, URGENCY URINARY INCONTINENCE, MIXED INCONTINENCE

1. Clinicians may perform multichannel filling cystometry when it is important to determine if altered compliance, DO, or other urodynamic abnormalities are present (or not) in patients with urgency incontinence in whom invasive, potentially morbid, or irreversible treatments are considered. (Option; Evidence Strength: Grade C)

A. Filling cystometry is the most precise way to obtain information relative to bladder storage. In patients with urinary storage symptoms, such as urgency and frequency, cystometry is the most appropriate way to assess storage and filling pressures.

B. Although UDS may not precisely predict outcomes of treatment, it may aide in symptom correlation in patients with mixed incontinence.[19,20]

C. If a patient has concomitant disorders, such as failed medical management of OAB, SUI, or BOO, identifying and treating these conditions could possibly improve patient outcome.

2. Clinicians may perform PFS in patients with urgency incontinence after bladder outlet procedures to evaluate for BOO. (Expert Opinion)

A. Patients who have undergone anti-incontinence procedures and have refractory OAB symptoms (with or without incontinence) may have these symptoms resulting

Table 3
Clinical case scenario 2 (POP)

77-y-Old with Chief Complaint of Vaginal Bulge	77-y-Old with Chief Complaint of Vaginal Bulge

History:
  Failed pessary × 3
  Denies SUI or urgency
  Denies difficulty emptying bladder
  Not sexually active
  S/p hysterectomy
  MI 2 y ago
	History:
	  Failed pessary × 3
	  Denies SUI, ++ urgency
	  + Moderate difficulty emptying bladder
	  Not sexually active
	  S/p hysterectomy
	  MI 2 y ago

Physical examination:
  Total prolapse
  Cuff at + 6
  POPQ Stage 4
  PVR 48 mL
	Physical examination:
	  Total prolapse
	  Cuff at + 6
	  POPQ Stage 4
	  PVR 48 mL

Recommendation:
  Stress test with prolapse reduction
	Recommendation:
	  UDS including pressure flow study with ALPP assessment after prolapse reduction

Discussion:
  In this scenario, this patient has no associated LUTS or SUI. If the decision has been reached to perform POP surgery because of bothersome prolapse symptoms, a stress test with the prolapse reduced will reveal whether patient is at significant risk for postoperative occult SUI. Multichannel UDS is optional if all of the necessary information has been obtained during this testing
	Discussion:
	  In this patient, there is associated storage symptoms such as urgency, and there are emptying LUTS as well. This complex constellation of symptoms may be better assessed with UDS, and the stress testing with prolapse reduction can be performed in this setting. Thus, all the desired information pertaining to LUTS and whether or not occult SUI will be obtained

Abbreviations: MI, myocardial infarction; POPQ, pelvic organ prolapse quantification; S/p, status post.

from BOO. Although there is no established urodynamic standard for women, elevated detrusor pressure and decreased flow are highly suggestive of BOO. This information could then be used to counsel patients regarding further treatment options.

   i. Consistent and perpetual elevated PVR after SUI surgery and significant change in LUTS after outlet procedure are so suggestive of BOO that UDS is likely unnecessary, and treatment of obstruction should be considered.

  B. It is reasonable to perform PFS on women with storage LUTS not responding to conservative treatments to rule out the possibility of BOO.

3. Clinicians should counsel patients with urgency incontinence and mixed incontinence that the absence of DO on a single urodynamic study does not exclude it as a causative agent for their symptoms. (Clinical Principle)

  A. The technical limitations of urodynamic tests do not allow for the detection of DO (the urodynamic finding of involuntary contractions of the bladder) in some patients, despite level of symptomatology. Because of these

limitations, it is recommended that testing be performed in such a way that symptoms be replicated as precisely as possible.

NEUROGENIC BLADDER

1. Clinicians should perform PVR assessment, either as part of complete urodynamic study or separately, during the initial urologic evaluation of patients with relevant neurologic conditions (eg, spinal cord injury, myelomeningocele) and as part of ongoing follow-up when appropriate. (Standard; Evidence Strength: Grade B)

  A. The Panel defines relevant neurologic conditions as those neurogenic disorders of lower urinary tract dysfunction that may predispose a patient to upper tract complications or renal impairment (**Table 4**).[21–23]

  B. Although PVR alone may not provide all the information necessary to make a treatment recommendation, it can be helpful in determining if further testing is indicated.

2. Clinicians should perform a complex cystometrogram (CMG) during initial urologic evaluation of patients with relevant neurologic conditions with or without symptoms and as part of

Table 4
Classification of common neurogenic lower urinary tract conditions by upper tract risk

Relevant NLUT Disorders (Risk of Upper Tract Complication)	Other NLUT Disorders (Little Risk of Upper Tract Complication)
Spinal cord injury	Parkinson disease
Transverse myelitis	Brain tumor
Myelomeningocele	Cerebrovascular accident
Radical pelvic surgery	Lumbar disc disease
Men with multiple sclerosis	Women with multiple sclerosis
Radical pelvic surgery	
Any NGB disorder with upper tract complications	

ongoing follow-up when appropriate. In patients with other neurologic diseases, physicians may consider CMG as an option in the urologic evaluation of patients with LUTS. (Recommendation; Evidence Strength: Grade C)

A. In patients presenting with neurogenic lower urinary tract (NLUT) disorders, patients with relevant conditions that may predispose them to upper tract risk should undergo a PFS (or cystometry if not voiding) despite whether or not they are having symptoms. In these patients, the initial study should be performed after the period of spinal shock has resolved. In these patients, the UDS is not only diagnostic but also prognostic.[23,24]

   i. In patients with relevant NLUT disorder with poor compliance or elevated detrusor leak point pressures on UDS, treatment needs to be directed at lowering urinary storage pressure even in the absence of symptoms.

   ii. Risks of infection and autonomic dysreflexia (AD) should be considered before proceeding with UDS in this patient population.

3. Clinicians should perform PFS in patients with relevant neurologic disease with or without symptoms or in patients with other neurologic disease and elevated PVR or urinary symptoms. (Recommendation; Evidence Strength: Grade C)

A. In patients with NLUT disorders that pose minimal upper tract risk, multichannel UDS (PFS or cystometry if not voiding) may be used selectively if there are symptoms or signs that suggest failure of empiric treatment, change in the bladder condition, or

that a more complicated clinical picture has evolved.

   i. Thus multichannel studies should be performed on any patient with NLUT disorder with any of the following conditions: elevated PVR, hydronephrosis, pyelonephritis, complicated urinary tract infections, or frequent episodes of AD.

   ii. Patients who continue to leak involuntarily between catheterizations may benefit from multichannel UDS.

   iii. Benign prostatic hyperplasia, OAB, and SUI can coexist in patients with neurogenic bladder (NGB). UDS may aid in diagnosis and may help guide potential therapy and monitor treatment outcomes.[25–27]

4. When available, clinicians may perform fluoroscopy at the time of UDS, VUDS, in patients with relevant neurologic disease at risk for NLUT dysfunction or in patients with other neurologic disease and elevated PVR or urinary symptoms. (Recommendation; Evidence Strength: Grade C)[23,28]

A. Benefits of fluoroscopy during UDS include the following:

   i. Delineating specific sites of obstruction (bladder neck or external sphincter)

   ii. Identifying the presence and grade of vesicoureteral reflux

      1. Identifying the urodynamic parameters that are present at the time of reflux

   iii. Identifying anatomic and physical abnormalities of the bladder and urethra.

B. Simultaneous fluoroscopy and cystometrogram and PFS provide more information than that gathered from performing each test separately.

5. Clinicians should perform EMG in combination with CMG with or without PFS in patients with relevant neurologic disease at risk for NGB or in patients with other neurologic disease and elevated PVR or urinary symptoms. (Recommendation; Evidence Strength: Grade C)[29,30]

A. The most important measurement provided by EMG testing is to determine whether perineal contractions are coordinated or uncoordinated with detrusor contractions. This testing modality is useful to assist in the diagnosis of detrusor external sphincter dyssynergia (DESD).

   i. The major limitation to EMG testing is its nonspecific nature, as EMG signals measure not only the external urethral sphincter but also the external anal sphincter and pelvic floor musculature. Needle electrodes may facilitate isolation of the urethral sphincter but require significant operator experience.

   ii. The EMG signals need to be taken in context of those gathered from fluoroscopy and UDS.

   iii. Benefits include the ability to diagnose DESD, which is characterized by involuntary contraction of external urethral sphincter during detrusor contraction (**Table 5**)

LOWER URINARY TRACT SYMPTOMS

For the purposes of the UDS Guideline, LUTS was confined to obstructive LUTS, because the role of UDS was examined in the area of storage LUTS in the section on urinary urgency and urgency incontinence.

1. Clinicians may perform PVR in patients with LUTS as a safety measure to rule out significant urinary retention both initially and during follow-up. (Clinical Principle)

   A. Most would agree that PVR measurement (particularly when done by ultrasonography) is a low-risk and minimally invasive assessment, which may be useful in screening patients with obstructive LUTS.

      i. This test may identify patients with significant urinary retention, and treatment is guided based on these findings along with the clinical assessment.

   B. PVR measurement is enhanced by more than 1 test, as the results may be variable. Treatment should not be guided by 1 PVR measurement alone.

   C. An elevation in PVR does not distinguish between BOO or impaired bladder contractility. Further testing (PFS) may be needed to make this distinction.

2. Uroflow may be used by clinicians in the initial and ongoing evaluation of men with LUTS that suggest an abnormality of voiding/emptying. (Recommendation; Evidence Strength: Grade C)

   A. Similar to PVR, uroflow represents a noninvasive screen of bladder emptying status. This test is also subject to significant artifact and may have great variability, but it may be useful during the initial evaluation and can monitor patients who have undergone treatment.[31,32]

   B. There are little data on the use of uroflow to provide guidance on its most appropriate use.

Table 5
Clinical case scenario 3 (NLUT dysfunction)

22-y-Old Man with Chief Complaint of Urinary Incontinence Between Catheterization	47-y-Old Woman with Chief Complaint of Urinary Urgency and Urgency Incontinence

History:
  Thoracic-level SCI
  Performs CIC 4–5 × daily
  Denies difficulty with catheterization
  + Incontinence between catheterization; no febrile UTIs
	History:
	  MS dx'd 4 y ago
	  No difficulty with emptying bladder
	  No UTIs or pyelonephritis
	  No prior surgery

Physical examination:
  Normal genitalia
  Spastic lower extremities
	Physical examination:
	  Normal genitalia
	  No prolapse

Recommendation:
  Videourodynamics
	Recommendation:
	  PVR followed by empiric therapy

Discussion:
  In this scenario, the patient has a spinal cord injury, which places him at significant risk for the development of upper tract complications if left unmanaged. This patient should undergo videourodynamics regardless of symptoms to evaluate his upper tract risk. In addition, the LUT dysfunction predisposing to leakage between catheterizations can be delineated as well
	Discussion:
	  In this scenario, this female patient has minimal risk to predispose to upper tract complications. In this setting, it is reasonable to screen with a PVR assessment and proceed to empiric therapy. An elevation in her PVR, nonresponse to therapy, or an intervening complication may warrant additional multichannel UDS tests. However, in this setting, screening and empiric treatment would be appropriate because of her minimal risk of upper tract complications

Abbreviations: CIC, clean intermittent catheterization; MS, multiple sclerosis; UTI, urinary tract infection.

3. Clinicians may perform multichannel filling cystometry when it is important to determine if DO or other abnormalities of bladder filling/urine storage are present in patients with LUTS, particularly when invasive, potentially morbid, or irreversible treatments are considered. (Expert Opinion)

   A. The panel still believes that in certain patients, the finding of significant DO or poor compliance on CMG could alter treatment recommendations or lead the physician to counsel the patient differently.

      i. Thus, the panel believes that in some patients, CMG is an acceptable diagnostic study for the evaluation of patients with LUTS.

4. Clinicians should perform PFS in men when it is important to determine if urodynamic obstruction is present in men with LUTS, particularly when invasive, potentially morbid, or irreversible treatments are considered. (Standard; Evidence Strength: Grade B)

   A. The use of PFS in men as a routine diagnostic test before elective surgery for benign prostatic enlargement remains a long-standing controversy. There are many studies that address this issue, and clearly the results are inconclusive. These answers are elusive as there are limitations in study design and variability of outcome measurement. Despite this, there are a significant number of trials demonstrating that PFS are predictive of outcomes after prostatectomy. The only definitive way to obtain a diagnosis of BOO is by PFS, which demonstrates high voiding pressure and low urinary flow.[33,34]

   B. There are also other concomitant findings (significant DO or poor compliance) that could alter treatment recommendations or lead the physician to counsel the patient differently before elective surgery.[35]

   C. It is clear that if the diagnosis is uncertain, or there is a complex presentation of LUTS in men, the only way to obtain an accurate diagnosis of obstruction is through PFS. In these patients, PFS should be performed.

   D. In other men presenting with uncomplicated obstructive LUTS, the only way to obtain urodynamic diagnosis of obstruction is by

Table 6
Clinical case scenario 4

67-y-Old Man with Chief Complaint of LUTS	37-y-Old Man with Chief Complaint of LUTS

Symptoms:
  + Weak stream and intermittent flow
    incomplete emptying urinary urgency
  Failed medical management
	Symptoms:
	  + Weak stream and intermittent flow
	    incomplete emptying urinary urgency
	  Failed medical management

Physical examination:
  Moderately enlarged prostate
	Physical examination:
	  Normal prostate

Diagnostics:
  Voided volume: 150 mL
  Maximum flow: 9 mL/s
  PVR: 130 mL
	Diagnostics:
	  Voided volume: 150 mL
	  Maximum flow: 9 mL/s
	  PVR: 130 mL

Recommendation:
  Surgery (TURP or equivalent outlet procedure)
	Recommendation:
	  VUDS and cystoscopy

Discussion:
  In this scenario, this gentleman has obstructive LUTS. His age, prostatic enlargement, and diagnostic studies strongly suggest (but do not definitively diagnose) obstruction. In this setting, proceeding to surgery is reasonable. Urodynamics is an option to evaluate for any other factors that may influence treatment or patient counseling
	Discussion:
	  In this scenario, there are several factors that represent a complicated setting of male LUTS. This patient's young age and his small prostatic size are not common in the presentation of male LUTS. In this setting, a diagnosis of obstruction should be sought (and the only way to obtain the diagnosis of obstruction is PFS). A cystoscopy should be considered to rule out anatomic abnormalities. Thus, in this complex scenario, PFS is recommended. VUDS should be considered to more precisely localize the level of obstruction

Abbreviation: TURP, transurethral resection of the prostate.

PFS. As discussed earlier, PVR and uroflow cannot determine if obstruction is present or not if interpreted alone. Thus, if a urodynamic diagnosis of obstruction is deemed necessary, the only way to do that is via PFS.

5. Clinicians may perform PFS in women when it is important to determine if obstruction is present. (Recommendation; Evidence Quality: Grade C)

A. Although studies have failed to correlate PFS findings with surgical outcome in women, the use of PFS is still considered beneficial in some women before intervention. In women with LUTS after anti-incontinence procedures or with significant obstructive symptoms, PFS may assist in obtaining the diagnosis of obstruction, which may influence management.[36,37]

B. The diagnosis of obstruction in women remains less straightforward than that in men, and PFS results should be taken in context with other clinical findings.[38,39]

6. Clinicians may perform VUDS in properly selected patients to localize the level of obstruction, particularly for diagnosing primary bladder neck obstruction (PBNO). (Expert Opinion)

A. VUDS evaluation (PFS with fluoroscopy) is useful in select women with LUTS. The use of VUDS is the only diagnostic tool that can document pressure/flow parameters and localize functional bladder-neck and external urethral sphincter anatomy. As such, these studies can differentiate between PBNO, dysfunctional voiding, and DESD.

i. Fluoroscopy is the only way to obtain the diagnosis of PBNO. The PFS findings of high voiding pressure and low urinary flow associated with radiographic confirmation of a nonrelaxing (closed) bladder neck during voiding are necessary to diagnose this rare condition (**Table 6**).

REFERENCES

1. Nager C, Brubaker L, Litman H, et al. A randomized trial of urodynamic testing before stress-incontinence surgery. N Engl J Med 2012;366:1987–97.

2. Monoski M, Gonzalez R, Sandhu J, et al. Urodynamic predictors of outcome with photoselective laser vaporization prostatectomy in patients with benign prostatic hyperplasia and preoperative retention. Urology 2006;68:312–7.

3. Djavan B, Madersbacher S, Klingler C, et al. Urodynamic assessment of patients with acute urinary retention: is treatment failure after prostatectomy predictable? J Urol 1997;158:1829–33.

4. Hosker G, Rosier P, Gajewski J, et al. Dynamic testing. In: Abrams P, Cardozo L, Khoury S, et al, editors. Incontinence. 4th edition. London: Health Publications Ltd; 2009. p. 413.

5. Scarpero H, Kaufman M, Koski M, et al. Urodynamics best practices. In: American Urological Association update series, vol. XXVIII, Lesson IX. 2009.

6. AUA methodology for guideline statements. Available at: http://www.auanet.org/education/standard-operating-procedures-overview.cfm. Accessed March 15, 2014.

7. Faraday M, Hubbard H, Kosiak B, et al. Staying at the cutting edge: a review and analysis of evidence reporting and grading: the recommendations of the American Urological Association. BJU Int 2009; 104:294.

8. Bunyavejchevin S. Can pre-operative urodynamic study predict the successful outcome of tension free vaginal tape (TVT) operation in Thai women with stress urinary incontinence? J Med Assoc Thai 2005;88:1493.

9. Kilicarslan H, Gokce G, Ayan S, et al. Predictors of outcome after in situ anterior vaginal wall sling surgery. Int Urogynecol J Pelvic Floor Dysfunct 2003;14:339.

10. Hsiao SM, Sheu BC, Lin HH. Sequential assessment of urodynamic findings before and after transobturator tape procedure for female urodynamic stress incontinence. Int Urogynecol J Pelvic Floor Dysfunct 2008;19:627.

11. Rechberger T, Futyma K, Jankiewicz K, et al. The clinical effectiveness of retropubic (IVS-02) and transobturator (IVS-04) midurethral slings: randomized trial. Eur Urol 2009;56:24–30.

12. Holtedahl K, Verelst M, Schiefloe A, et al. Usefulness of urodynamic examination in female urinary incontinence–lessons from a population-based, randomized, controlled study of conservative treatment. Scand J Urol Nephrol 2000;34:169.

13. Dmochowski RR, Blaivas JM, Gormley EA, et al. Female stress urinary incontinence update panel of the American Urological Association Education and Research, Inc. Update of AUA guideline on the surgical management of female stress urinary incontinence. J Urol 2010;183:1906.

14. Maniam P, Goldman HB. Removal of transurethral catheter during urodynamics may unmask stress urinary incontinence. J Urol 2002;167:2080.

15. Huckabay C, Twiss C, Berger A, et al. A urodynamics protocol to optimally assess men with post-prostatectomy incontinence. Neurourol Urodyn 2005;24:622.

16. Mueller ER, Kenton K, Mahajan S, et al. Urodynamic prolapse reduction alters urethral pressure but not filling or pressure flow parameters. J Urol 2007; 177:600.

17. Visco AG, Brubaker L, Nygaard I, et al. Pelvic Floor Disorders Network: the role of preoperative urodynamic testing in stress-continent women undergoing sacrocolpopexy: the Colpopexy and Urinary Reduction Efforts (CARE) randomized surgical trial. Int Urogynecol J Pelvic Floor Dysfunct 2008;19:607.

18. Araki I, Haneda Y, Mikami Y, et al. Incontinence and detrusor dysfunction associated with pelvic organ prolapse: clinical value of preoperative urodynamic evaluation. Int Urogynecol J Pelvic Floor Dysfunct 2009;20:1301.

19. Lee KS, Choo MS, Doo CK, et al. The long term (5-years) objective TVT success rate does not depend on predictive factors at multivariate analysis: a multicentre retrospective study. Eur Urol 2008;53:176.

20. Paick JS, Ku JH, Kim SW, et al. Tension-free vaginal tape procedure for the treatment of mixed urinary incontinence: significance of maximal urethral closure pressure. J Urol 2004;172:1001.

21. Araki I, Matsui M, Ozawa K, et al. Relationship of bladder dysfunction to lesion site in multiple sclerosis. J Urol 2003;169:1384.

22. Sakakibara R, Kanda T, Sekido T, et al. Mechanism of bladder dysfunction in idiopathic normal pressure hydrocephalus. Neurourol Urodyn 2008;27:507.

23. Sakakibara R, Hattori T, Uchiyama T, et al. Videourodynamic and sphincter motor unit potential analyses in Parkinson's disease and multiple system atrophy. J Neurol Neurosurg Psychiatry 2001;71:600.

24. Nitti VW, Adler H, Combs AJ. The role of urodynamics in the evaluation of voiding dysfunction in men after cerebrovascular accident. J Urol 1996;155:263.

25. Natsume O. Detrusor contractility and overactive bladder in patients with cerebrovascular accident. Int J Urol 2008;15:505.

26. Kaplan SA, Te AE, Blaivas JG. Urodynamic findings in patients with diabetic cystopathy. J Urol 1995;153:342.

27. Rapidi CA, Karandreas N, Katsifotis C, et al. A combined urodynamic and electrophysiological study of diabetic cystopathy. Neurourol Urodyn 2006;25:32.

28. Light JK, Beric A, Petronic I. Detrusor function with lesions of the cauda equina, with special emphasis on the bladder neck. J Urol 1993;149:539.

29. Ciancio SJ, Mutchnik SE, Rivera VM, et al. Urodynamic pattern changes in multiple sclerosis. Urology 2001;57:239.

30. Rovner E, Wein A. Practical urodynamics. In: American Urological Association update series. vol. 21. 2002. p. 19.

31. Aganovic D. The role of uroflowmetry in diagnosis of infravesical obstruction in the patients with benign prostatic enlargement. Med Arh 2004;58:109.

32. Comiter CV, Sullivan MP, Schacterle RS, et al. Prediction of prostatic obstruction with a combination of isometric detrusor contraction pressure and maximum urinary flow rate. Urology 1996; 48:723.

33. Thomas AW, Cannon A, Bartlett E, et al. The natural history of lower urinary tract dysfunction in men: minimum 10-year urodynamic follow-up of transurethral resection of prostate for bladder outlet obstruction. J Urol 2005;174:1887.

34. Van Venrooij GE, Van Melick HH, Eckhardt MD, et al. Correlations of urodynamic changes with changes in symptoms and well-being after transurethral resection of the prostate. J Urol 2002;168:605.

35. Cho MC, Kim HS, Lee CJ, et al. Influence of detrusor overactivity on storage symptoms following potassium-titanyl-phosphate photoselective vaporization of the prostate. Urology 2010;75:1460.

36. Basu M, Duckett J. The effect of urethral dilatation on pressure flow studies in women with voiding dysfunction and overactive bladder. Int Urogynecol J Pelvic Floor Dysfunct 2009;20:1073.

37. Kobak WH, Walters MD, Piedmonte MR. Determinants of voiding after three types of incontinence surgery: a multivariable analysis. Obstet Gynecol 2001;97:86.

38. Defreitas GA, Zimmern PE, Lemack GE, et al. Refining diagnosis of anatomic female bladder outlet obstruction: comparison of pressure-flow study parameters in clinically obstructed women with those of normal control. Urology 2004;64: 675.

39. Blaivas JG, Groutz A. Bladder outlet obstruction nomogram for women with lower urinary tract symptomatology. Neurourol Urodyn 2000;19:553.

Good Urodynamic Practice
Keys to Performing A Quality UDS Study

Lara S. MacLachlan, MD, Eric S. Rovner, MD*

KEYWORDS

- Urodynamics • Videourodynamics • Transducer catheters • Plausibility • Artifacts

KEY POINTS

- The clinician should identify the clinical questions that the urodynamics (UDS) study is intended to answer, properly design the study to answer those questions, and be able to adapt the study as necessary.
- The UDS study should be performed interactively and with continuous communication with the patient to confirm that their symptoms have been reproduced.
- Careful observation of signals is important to assess their qualitative and quantitative plausibility, such that artifacts can be recognized and corrected during the study.
- The quality and results of the UDS study are operator-dependent and are only as good as the clinician who performs and interprets the study.
- A well-done UDS study may be invaluable in the diagnosis of lower urinary tract conditions, or assessing prognosis and response to therapy, or directing management; however, a poorly done study may be misleading and potentially harmful.

INTRODUCTION

Urodynamics (UDS) is a collection of measurements of bladder, urethral, and pelvic floor muscle function with or without fluoroscopy (videourodynamics or VUDS) in an attempt to evaluate and diagnose functional, and sometimes anatomic, disorders of the lower urinary tract. The goal of performing UDS studies in many cases is to reproduce a patient's lower urinary tract symptoms while making precise measurements to identify the underlying causes for their symptoms.[1] In other cases, UDS are performed to assess prognosis or the results of prior therapy or to direct optimal therapy. UDS studies are invasive, uncomfortable, and potentially morbid. It is therefore imperative to optimize the quality of the study to maximize the useful information that can be obtained. When possible, UDS should be performed interactively with the patient, which includes confirmation with the patient throughout the study that their symptoms or conditions have been reproduced during the test.

COMPONENTS OF UDS

UDS comprises different components that can be used individually or collectively to gain information about urine storage and evacuation. In performing a quality study, a working knowledge of each component and their role is important to understand.

Postvoid Residual

Postvoid residual (PVR) is an assessment of bladder emptying and can be performed by ultrasound/ bladder scan or catheterization. An elevated PVR

Disclosures: None.
Department of Urology, Medical University of South Carolina, 96 Jonathan Lucas Street, CSB 644, Charleston, SC 29425, USA
* Corresponding author.
E-mail address: rovnere@musc.edu

Urol Clin N Am 41 (2014) 363–373
http://dx.doi.org/10.1016/j.ucl.2014.04.005

can be an indication of a bladder-emptying problem, but cannot distinguish the cause of the problem, such as bladder outlet obstruction (BOO) or detrusor underactivity or a combination of both. PVR can be assessed using ultrasound, either in real-time or by portable bladder scan, or via catheterization. In obese patients or those with ascites, or prior lower abdominal surgery, bladder scan is inaccurate and real-time ultrasound or catheterization is preferred.[2,3]

Uroflowmetry

Uroflowmetry is a noninvasive measurement of the rate of urine flow over time. It can also be used to assess bladder emptying but cannot be used alone to diagnose the cause of an abnormality. For example, a low maximum flow and plateaued pattern on uroflowmetry cannot distinguish between BOO and impaired detrusor contractility. Other patterns are easily recognized but are also not completely diagnostic: a superflow pattern implies decreased urethral closure forces but may be due to volitional abdominal straining, whereas a saw-toothed pattern suggests Valsalva voiding but may be due to intermittent voluntary or involuntary contraction of the external sphincter or pelvic floor (**Fig. 1**). It is imperative in all circumstances to query the patient as to whether their usual voiding pattern or behavior was accurately reflected on the noninvasive uroflowmetry study.

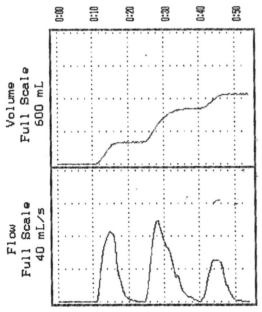

Fig. 1. Uroflowmetry pattern suggestive of Valsalva voiding or pelvic floor dysfunction.

The most commonly used uroflowmeters are mass flow meters, such as those that use a gravimetric method or a rotating disc method. Uroflowmeters that use a gravimetric meter operate by measuring the accumulated weight of the collected fluid or by measuring the hydrostatic pressure at the bottom of a collection cylinder. Rotating disc instruments use the voided fluid directly on a rotating disc to increase the inertia of the disc. The power required to keep the disc rotating at a constant rate is measured and is proportional to the mass flow rate of the fluid.[4]

Filling Cystometry

Filling cystometry is a measurement of the pressure/volume relationship during bladder filling. It is performed using measurements of intravesical pressure (Pves) and intra-abdominal pressure (Pabd) to calculate the detrusor pressure (Pdet = Pves – Pabd). The key features of bladder storage function obtainable with filling cystometry include sensation, cystometric bladder capacity, compliance, and presence of involuntary detrusor contractions or detrusor overactivity (DO).[5] Leak point pressures, an assessment of urethral function, are also assessed during filling cystometry. These features will be discussed in greater detail later.

Pressure-Flow Study

The relationship between bladder pressure and urine flow rate is measured during bladder emptying.[6] The pressure-flow study is currently the only method of diagnosing BOO and/or impaired detrusor contractility (or detrusor underactivity). There are 3 fundamental voiding states that can be diagnosed by the pressure-flow study, which include obstruction, impaired detrusor contractility, and normal.[5] During the pressure-flow urodynamic study (PFUD), several parameters are assessed: detrusor contractility, coordination of the detrusor and outlet, bladder emptying, and the presence or absence of UDS obstruction.

Electromyography

Electromyography (EMG) is the measurement of the electrical signals produced by the depolarization of muscle membranes.[6] EMG studies can be performed using either surface electrodes or needle EMG, which is more invasive, to measure electrical activity from the pelvic floor muscles. EMG is measured throughout the UDS study during both the filling and the emptying phases. The EMG tracing is used to assess the coordination or discoordination of the external urethral sphincter and the detrusor contraction.

Fluoroscopy

When the UDS study is combined with an imaging modality, the anatomy and physiology of the lower urinary tract can be simultaneously assessed, which is referred to as VUDS. The use of fluoroscopy provides anatomic information about the bladder, bladder neck, and urethra during filling and voiding that could not otherwise be obtained during the study without fluoroscopy. This portion of the study is useful for assessing for vesicoureteral reflux (VUR) as well.

Fluoroscopic images may be obtained at various points throughout the study. Before starting the study, a scout film is obtained to identify any surgical hardware or bladder stones before the contrast-filled bladder obscures them. Images can be captured during early bladder filling to assess the contour of the bladder and identify any possible filling defects. Next, a sequence of images taken at rest and then during abdominal strain/Valsalva maneuvers is used to assess mobility of the bladder base, bladder neck, and urethra as well as the competence of the bladder outlet and urethra. Multiple fluoroscopic images taken during voiding can evaluate the bladder neck and urethra as well as document the presence or absence of VUR. Images of the bladder and the upper tracts (kidneys, ureter, bladder, flat plate x-ray [KUB]) can be obtained to assess VUR, bladder or urethral diverticula, and other potential pathologic abnormalities. Because most VUDS studies are done in the seated position using a C-arm apparatus for imaging, anterior-posterior imaging is most commonly used. However, there are instances where oblique or lateral images are superior, such as when assessing for bladder diverticula, cystocele, and urethral stricture.[7]

PRETEST CONSIDERATIONS

To perform a quality UDS study, the clinician must identify the clinical questions that the UDS study is intended to answer before any testing is performed. To do so, the clinician needs a working knowledge of the patient's history, physical examination findings, frequency/volume charts, and any other information to identify clinical relevant findings during the UDS study.[5] A bladder diary performed before the UDS study that records voided volumes can be used to correlate the patient's bladder diary capacity to the cystometric capacity obtained during the study. These capacities should be plausibly similar to appropriately reproduce the patient's symptoms. Pad testing can be used to quantify the amount of urine lost during incontinence episodes, which can provide valuable information before the UDS study. Small amounts of leakage can suggest stress urinary incontinence, whereas large amounts of leakage can be suggestive of urge urinary incontinence. For the incontinent patient, either of these conditions may be demonstrated; however, it is paramount to relate the condition seen on UDS study to the patient's primary complaint to ensure that the symptoms, or condition, are reproduced by the finding on the UDS study.

The clinician should design the UDS study to answer the clinical questions and customize the study as needed. For example, in a patient who complains of symptoms of mixed urinary incontinence, the test may be conducted to assess for the predominant type of incontinence. Reproduction of the patient's incontinence is critically important, especially to the extent that it reproduces the patient's symptoms. In such a patient, stress maneuvers, change in positioning, or provocative maneuvers (hand washing and so on) may be necessary to induce the symptoms. In contrast, for the patient with neurogenic voiding dysfunction in which potential compliance issues are most important, such maneuvers are unnecessary and even counterproductive. In the patient with vaginal prolapse, a repeat study with a pessary may be needed (see later discussion). In the patient with possible BOO, every effort should be made to produce a detrusor contraction because the voiding phase of the UDS study is likely the most relevant. BOO cannot be definitively diagnosed without a detrusor contraction. Sometimes, in those individuals with difficulty initiating a void, a detrusor contraction might be induced by a change in position or a rapid filling rate.

In deciding when to perform a VUDS over a UDS study, the clinician should consider whether obtaining simultaneous fluoroscopic images would improve the ability to detect and understand the underlying pathologic abnormalities, such as specific sites of obstruction, presence and grade of VUR, and anatomic abnormalities of the bladder. The American Urological Association (AUA) Guidelines for Adult Urodynamics recommends that VUDS be performed in patients with relevant neurologic disease who are at risk for neurogenic bladder, or in patients with other neurologic disease and elevated PVR or urinary symptoms.[8] The AUA Update Series on Urodynamics Best Practices recommends that VUDS be performed in those patients at high risk for voiding dysfunction, such as those with known or suspected neurogenic bladder, prior radical pelvic surgery, urinary diversion, renal transplant, or prior pelvic radiation.[5] Further discussion about indications and techniques for performing VUDS is covered elsewhere in this issue.

For the safety of the patient, it should be confirmed that the patient is not experiencing a urinary tract infection (UTI) before the UDS study.[5] For those patients who perform intermittent catheterization or have indwelling catheters, it may not be possible to sterilize the urine before the UDS study, but it is important to ensure that the patient is asymptomatic to differentiate between bacterial colonization and active infection. If the patient is experiencing a UTI, then the UDS study should be postponed until the patient is free of infection.

Finally, before the UDS study, patients should be well informed about why the test is being done and what to expect during the actual UDS test. Providing reassurances to the patient before the start of the study can reduce anxiety felt by the patient.[9]

PERFORMING THE STUDY

Positioning of the patient for the UDS study should account for the patient's functional status, the symptoms that the clinician would like to reproduce, and the patient's normal voiding habits. If the patient only experiences urinary incontinence while in the standing position, then the filling portion of the study should be performed with the patient standing. If a patient only voids while sitting, then the voiding portion of the study should be performed with the patient in the seated position. To obtain the best study results, the goal is to make the testing experience as close to the patient's normal voiding experience as possible.

UDS pressure measurements are obtained via a transducer catheter, which converts pressure into an electrical signal that is displayed as a tracing.[10] There are many different types of transducers, which include air-charged, fluid-filled, microtransducers, and fiberoptic systems. The International Continence Society (ICS) recommends fluid-filled transducers to be used for Pves and Pabd recordings.[1] For simultaneous measurement of intravesical pressure and for bladder filling, the ICS recommends a transurethral double-lumen catheter. For the measurement of abdominal pressures, the ICS recommends the use of a rectal balloon catheter with the balloon only filled to 10% to 20% of its unstretched capacity.[1] In female patients, placement of the rectal catheter in the posterior vaginal vault is an acceptable alternative that provides comparable results.

UDS catheters should be zeroed to atmospheric pressure before insertion, and the ICS recommends strict adherence to its standardization of zero pressure and standard height.[1,5] Zero pressure is defined as the value recorded when a transducer that is disconnected from any tubes or catheters is open to the environment, or when the open end of a fluid-filled tube is at the same level as the transducer.[1] The ICS defines the reference height as the upper edge of the symphysis pubis.

UDS catheters are inherently uncomfortable during placement except in patients who are insensate or who are on regular intermittent catheterization. Such discomfort with catheter placement can result in artifacts during the study, especially abnormal sensation of filling, as well as suppression of normal micturition. In some individuals, placement of intraurethral topical lidocaine jelly may reduce discomfort associated with catheterization and thereby alleviate some anxiety about the procedure as well as facilitate voiding by reducing the catheter-associated dysuria. Whether such administration of topical anesthetic changes bladder sensation with filling and thus alters the qualitative or quantitative results and findings of the study is unclear.

Filling and Storage

The patient should be instructed to void before the start of the UDS study in a private bathroom. On entry into the UDS room, and under sterile conditions, the patient is catheterized per urethra and the bladder is emptied before the start of the study, providing an accurate assessment of PVR. The catheters are placed and the filling phase then commences.

Throughout the study, the clinician should maintain continuous communication with the patient to confirm that their symptoms have been reproduced. In addition, the clinician should be carefully observing the signals to assess their qualitative and quantitative plausibility. When the quantitative result of a UDS study appears very abnormal or does not represent a plausible result in that particular clinical setting, alternative considerations should be considered.[11] The study should also be adjusted or repeated if the clinician cannot at first answer the questions that were posed at the start of the study.[5] It may be necessary to perform provocative maneuvers, which the ICS has defined as techniques used during UDS in an effort to provoke DO, such as rapid filling, use of cooled or acid medium, postural changes, and hand washing.[12]

Fill Rate and Capacity

When choosing a fill rate, the clinician needs to be aware that a standard fill rate cannot be applied to every patient. A fill rate that is too rapid can induce involuntary detrusor contractions, the appearance of impaired compliance, or an artifactually low cystometric bladder capacity. For children, patients with neurogenic bladder or urinary diversion, anuric patients, or patients with known small capacity bladders, a slower fill rate is preferred. Generally, a starting fill rate of 50 to 70 mL/min is acceptable for the adult patient because it minimizes artifact yet allows the study to be completed in a reasonable amount of time.[5]

Appropriate filling volumes should be attained to facilitate micturition and should be representative of the patient's normal circumstances. Therefore, it is helpful to have a frequency volume chart (or the more comprehensive voiding diary) before the UDS study to have an estimate of functional bladder capacity.

Sensation

Bladder sensation is judged by 3 defined points during the filling cystometry and is evaluated in relation to the bladder volume at that moment and in relation to the patient's symptomatic complaints.[12] The 3 sensory landmarks associated with performing a filling cystometry are first sensation of bladder filling, first desire to void, and strong desire to void. The ICS defines first sensation of bladder filling as the feeling when the patient first becomes aware of bladder filling. First desire to void is defined as the need to pass urine at the next convenient moment, but voiding can be delayed if necessary. Strong desire to void is defined as the persistent desire to void without the fear of leakage.[12] The patient should be instructed on each of these 3 sensory landmarks and reminded to report each sensation at regular intervals throughout the filling study.

Leak Point Pressure Testing

Abdominal leak point pressure (ALPP), also known as the Valsalva leak point pressure, is defined as the lowest intravesical pressure at which urine leakage occurs because of increased abdominal pressure in the absence of a detrusor contraction.[12] The ALPP can be used as an assessment of urethral competence and documentation of leak point pressures establishes the diagnosis of UDS stress urinary incontinence. ALPP should be distinguished from a detrusor leak point pressure (DLPP), which is defined as the lowest detrusor pressure at which urine leakage occurs in the absence of either a detrusor contraction or increased abdominal pressure.[12] DLPP is not used to directly measure continence or sphincter function, but is a useful parameter for assessing risk to the upper urinary tract as a result of elevated storage pressures.[13]

ALPP Testing

Although universal guidelines do not exist for the performance of ALPP across UDS laboratories, such testing should be standardized in each individual center so as to obtain reproducible and internally usable quantitative assessments of urethral function. Such testing should be done with a standard size and type of urethral catheter (usually dual lumen 7–8 Fr), in a standard position (sitting, standing, and so on), at a standard volume (150 cc, 200 cc, capacity, and so on), with a standard set of maneuvers (cough, Valsalva, graded or not, and so on). The ALPP measurement should never be performed at the time of an involuntary detrusor contraction, resulting in an artifactually low assessment of urethral function.

In patients with vaginal prolapse, reduction of the prolapse may be necessary to accurately assess the ALPP, as well as completely assess related voiding phase dysfunction later in the study. In such individuals, it can be instructive to perform the entire UDS study with and without the vaginal prolapse appropriately reduced with a pessary or vaginal packing.

In some patients, an ALPP may not be apparent during the study despite multiple attempts to produce it. In such cases, it may be helpful to remove the vesical catheter from the urethra, leaving the abdominal catheter in situ, and repeat testing using the abdominal catheter for the pressure measurement.

DLPP Testing

DLPP was initially described as a method to predict risk for upper urinary tract deterioration as a result of increased lower urinary tract storage pressures in myelodysplastic children.[13] For those patients with decreased bladder compliance and urinary incontinence as a result of neurogenic bladder dysfunction, DLPP testing can be a useful tool to assess risk to the upper urinary tract. A DLPP greater than 40 cm H_2O is considered hazardous to the upper tracts, whereas patients with a DLPP less than 40 cm H_2O commonly do not experience upper urinary tract deterioration in the absence of other complicating factors such as infection or VUR. However, some individuals may experience upper tract deterioration at DLPP at somewhat less than 40 cm H_2O and thus monitoring of such patients should be strongly considered.

Compliance

Compliance describes the relationship between change in bladder volume and change in detrusor pressure and is calculated by dividing the volume change by the change in detrusor pressure during that change in bladder volume.[12] The ICS recommends that the 2 standard points used to calculate compliance should be at the start of bladder filling and then at cystometric capacity or immediately before the start of any detrusor contraction that causes significant leakage. Normal compliance should be greater than 12.5 mL/cm H_2O.[5]

In patients at risk for upper urinary tract deterioration as a result of increased lower urinary tract storage pressure, compliance should be assessed carefully. Rapid bladder filling, infection, or long-standing indwelling catheter may be associated with an artifactually impaired compliance. A prolonged involuntary bladder contraction can also be misinterpreted as impaired compliance. In those patients with apparent impaired compliance on UDS testing, bladder filling should be stopped and the intravesical pressure examined to distinguish between impaired compliance (Pdet will remain elevated) and a prolonged involuntary detrusor contraction (Pdet will eventually return to near baseline). Finally, high-volume VUR or decompression into a large bladder diverticulum will result in artifactually low filling pressures and an overestimate of bladder compliance in patients who are at risk.

Involuntary Detrusor Contractions (DO)

DO is a UDS observation characterized by involuntary detrusor contractions during the filling phase, which may be spontaneous or provoked. Phasic detrusor overactivity is a pattern of DO defined by a characteristic waveform and may or may not lead to urinary incontinence. Per the ICS standardization documents, there is no lower limit to the amplitude that defines DO, but confident interpretation of low-pressure waves of less than 5 cm H_2O depends on "high-quality" UDS technique.[12] DO may occur during the filling portion of the study, which may or may not be suppressible. In fact, the ICS has updated the definition of DO so that it no longer includes the statement "involuntary detrusor contraction which the patient cannot completely suppress."[12] A single involuntary detrusor contraction that occurs at cystometric capacity, which cannot be suppressed and results in incontinence and bladder emptying, is termed terminal detrusor overactivity. An "after contraction" is a phasic increase in Pdet of significant amplitude, which occurs at the end of micturition with an empty bladder. The significance of such a contraction is unclear and may represent artifact from catheter malpositioning or true lower urinary tract pathologic abnormality.

Overall, the finding of DO may be clinically relevant or not. In patients without complaints of frequency, urgency, or urgency urinary incontinence, the finding of DO may be artifactual and irrelevant if it does not reproduce any of the patient's clinical symptoms. In such individuals, DO may be found in 14% to 18%.[14,15] In contrast, up to 50% of women with complaints of overactive bladder, symptoms with urgency incontinence will not demonstrate DO on UDS studies.[6] Provocative maneuvers, such as hand washing, and changes in position may induce DO in those individuals in whom it is suspected but not demonstrated.

Emptying

Micturition is typically a private activity for most patients, so reproducing normal voiding habits in a clinical UDS laboratory can be challenging. It is essential to create an environment that promotes privacy and maximal comfort for the patient in this highly unusual setting. In order for the UDS study to adequately answer the clinical questions, the patient should be instructed to void as they normally void at home, despite the artificial clinical setting. Patients should be questioned on whether the void during the UDS study reproduces their usual voiding pattern at home. For example, if the patient states that they push or strain during urination, then the UDS clinician should ensure that the voiding portion of the UDS study reflects that pattern. Alternatively, a straining pattern on the voiding portion of the UDS study that does not reproduce the patient's usual voiding habit is of minimal diagnostic value. A prestudy noninvasive uroflowmetry can be used to compare with the pressure-flow study of the UDS to ensure that they approximate each other. If not, the UDS clinician must decide which best represents the patient's voiding pattern and which is artifactual.

Many patients find that initiating a void during the UDS study extraordinarily difficult. Some of these factors may be environmental, such as attempting to void in front of others, with a catheter in the urethra, under fluoroscopy (in the setting of VUDS), and so on. Some patients have pain with urination and the anticipation of the pain, especially with a urethral catheter in place, may inhibit patients from voiding during the study. Other patients may have a long-standing history of "bashful bladder" or psychogenic inhibition, which is a condition characterized by the inability to initiate or maintain micturition in situations where there is a perception of scrutiny by others.[16] Reducing the number of personnel in the UDS laboratory during the study, the use of privacy screens, and the use of a "white noise" generator or playing relaxing music are maneuvers that can help reduce the "clinical" environment of the UDS laboratory and consequently help the patient feel more relaxed. Hearing running water from the sink faucet or bathing the patient's hands in warm water can help a patient initiate micturition. There are times when it may be necessary to have all the personnel leave the UDS laboratory and monitor the study remotely, or returning only after the patient has begun voiding.[17] Despite all of these maneuvers, there will be some patients who will still be unable to void. In this scenario, the intravesical catheter can be removed and the patient asked to void again in case the urethral catheter was preventing the patient from voiding (whether it be from an anatomic obstruction or from psychogenic inhibition). Data from Pves would be lost, but uroflowmetry combined with the Pabd tracing and fluoroscopic images if performing VUDS can be informative. If this fails, then all transducers and EMG patches/needles should be removed and the patient should be asked to void for a noninvasive uroflowmetry. If the patient is still unable to void for a noninvasive uroflowmetry, then a PVR measurement should be performed.

Obstruction

BOO is the generic term for obstruction diagnosed on a pressure-flow study during voiding and is characterized by a high detrusor pressure and a low flow rate.[12] The ICS recognizes that BOO has been defined for men but as of yet has not been adequately defined for women and children. Also, the diagnosis of BOO can only be made during UDS in the setting of a detrusor contraction. Thus, BOO cannot be diagnosed in the setting of a Valsalva void. However, other clinical entities can mimic BOO during a pressure-flow study, such as dysfunctional voiding, unrecognized pelvic organ prolapse, or pelvic floor/external sphincter spasm secondary to pain from catheterization. It is therefore important to recognize these clinical scenarios during a UDS study to prevent a misdiagnosis of BOO.

Coordination

Normal micturition begins with a relaxation of the bladder outlet and external sphincter followed by a detrusor contraction of adequate magnitude and duration to empty the bladder. The outlet should remain open until satisfactory bladder emptying is completed. Failure of the sphincter to relax or stay completely relaxed during micturition is considered abnormal.[6] Causes of incomplete coordination of the external sphincter and the detrusor muscle include detrusor sphincter

dyssynergia (DSD), dysfunctional voiding, and pain from the catheterization during the UDS study. DSD is defined as a detrusor contraction concurrent with an involuntary contraction of the urethral and/or periurethral striated muscle.[12] It is caused by a neurologic lesion in the suprasacral spinal cord and true DSD can only occur when there is a known neurologic lesion above the sacral micturition center. If there is no neurologic lesion, then the lack of coordination is considered to be a learned behavior known as dysfunctional voiding. It is characterized by an intermittent and/or fluctuating flow rate caused by involuntary intermittent contractions of the pelvic floor striated muscles during voiding in neurologically normal individuals.[12] The disorder is well described in children, but can be seen in adult men and women complaining of lower urinary tract symptoms. When diagnosing dysfunctional voiding on UDS studies, a noninvasive uroflowmetry should be performed for comparison to rule-out a test-induced phenomenon such as pain from the urethral catheter.[6]

Contractility

Bladder contractility depends on several factors, including pharmacologic, neurologic, smooth muscle, and others. Appropriate filling volumes should be attained to facilitate micturition. Underfilling or overfilling during UDS will result in an underestimation of detrusor contractility. Therefore, it is helpful to have a voiding diary before the UDS study to have an estimate of functional bladder capacity.

Normal detrusor function during voiding is defined as a voluntarily initiated continuous detrusor contraction that leads to complete bladder emptying within a normal time span, and in the absence of obstruction.[12] Abnormal detrusor activity can be subdivided into detrusor underactivity and acontractile detrusor. Detrusor underactivity is defined as a contraction of reduced strength and/or duration, resulting in prolonged bladder emptying and/or a failure to achieve complete bladder emptying within a normal time span.[12] If bladder contractility cannot be demonstrated during the UDS study, then it is considered an acontractile detrusor. Such a diagnosis of detrusor acontractility should not be applied unless the patient's voiding pattern during the UDS study is representative of the patient's usual voiding pattern and is confirmed not to be caused by the environmental circumstances of the study. These 2 states of abnormal bladder contractility can occur for various reasons including neurologic conditions and diabetes. However, pain from catheterization or psychogenic inhibition (bashful bladder) may result in temporary suppression of the micturition reflex and an apparent diminished contractility. A diagnosis of abnormal detrusor activity should not be applied unless the patient's voiding pattern, as reflected by detrusor acontractility, is representative of their usual voiding pattern at home and is confirmed not to be caused by the environmental circumstances of the study.

ARTIFACT RECOGNITION

It is important to understand that PFUDs are performed under very abnormal conditions. It is an attempt to reproduce a very private event (urinary filling and voiding) under nonphysiological and very public conditions. The filling medium is not isotonic with urine; it is infused at a nonphysiological rate and temperature, through an indwelling catheter in the company of other individuals. This event introduces considerable potential artifact. Filling fluid should be infused at a reasonable filling rate as described above. The filling fluid may be warmed to near body temperature. One of the more common issues encountered during a UDS study is that of psychogenic inhibition when a patient is unable to void normally when asked to do so during the study. Techniques to help relax the patient include playing relaxing music, limiting the staff members in the room, and running water in the sink. At times, it may be necessary to step out of the examination room and monitor the study

remotely or quickly return when the patient has begun voiding to capture the information needed.[17]

Artifacts during a UDS study can be either physiologic or technical in nature. When a physiologic event occurs that transiently affects the accuracy of one or more pressure measurements, it is considered a physiologic artifact.[10] A common physiologic artifact is a result of rectal contractions that cause an increase in abdominal pressure without an increase in intravesical pressure (Fig. 2), resulting in a spurious decline in detrusor pressure. A variety of technical artifacts can occur during UDS testing and are largely due to equipment failure, such as a kink in the intravesical catheter. Artifacts should be recognized early and corrected immediately.

Coughs are used to confirm that the intravesical and abdominal catheters are transmitting adequately and that the pressures are responding equally. The ICS recommends performing a cough test every 1 minute or 50 mL of infused volume.[1] These repeated assessments of pressure signals are especially important for those patients at increased risk of artifacts, which includes women with pelvic organ prolapse, morbidly obese patients, and following repositioning from the seated or standing position.[10] Breathing or talking may cause minor variations in the intravesical and abdominal pressures, but these should be similar for both pressures and not reflected in the detrusor pressure.

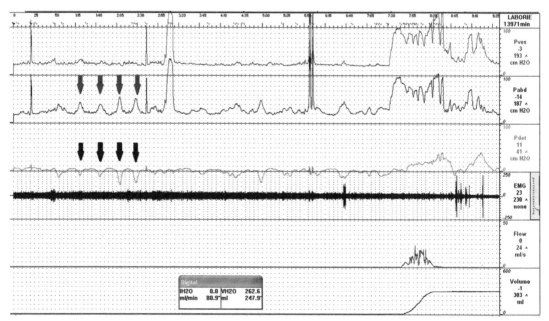

Fig. 2. Rectal contractions. A rise in Pabd (*red arrows*) without a rise in Pves, caused by rectal contractions, results in a spurious decline in Pdet (*black arrows*).

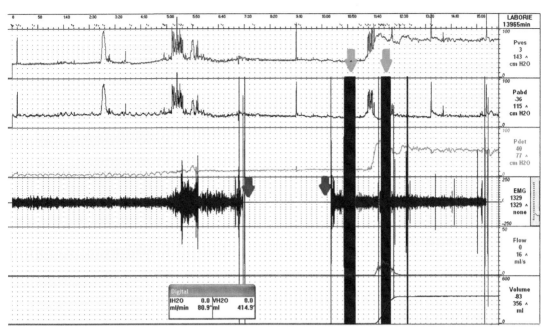

Fig. 3. All of the EMG leads lose contact, causing loss of EMG signal (between *red arrows*). Flaring of EMG signal because of loss of one EMG lead (*green arrows*).

Increases in abdominal pressures caused by Valsalva or coughing should be reflected in the intravesical pressure such that the 2 signals are mirror images of each other. When the signals from Pabd and Pves do not mirror each other, the clinician should be concerned for a signal mismatch. Common causes for signal mismatch

include problems with tubing connections, air in the tubing of a water-filled system, failure to charge an air-charged system, or positioning problems with the catheters.

EMG is susceptible to technical artifacts that can result in erroneous electrical activity on the EMG. Any electrical device operating near the

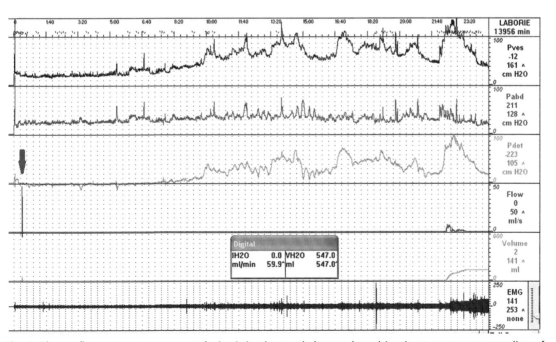

Fig. 4. The uroflowmetry measurement device is inadvertently bumped resulting in an erroneous recording of the urinary flow rate and voided volume (*red arrow*).

UDS system that has the potential to create a 60-cycle line voltage can be a source of EMG artifact.[18] Improper grounding or placement of electrodes can also produce an inaccurate EMG signal. Other common sources of EMG artifact is when voiding across a patch electrode causes it to become wet and when a patch loses adherence to the skin (**Fig. 3**).

Artifacts occurring during uroflowmetry should be immediately recognized and corrected when possible. A common artifact is when the uroflowmetry measurement device is inadvertently bumped, resulting in an erroneous recording of the urinary flow rate and voided volume (**Fig. 4**), and in a very recognizable sharp spike on the flow signal line. Another common uroflowmetry artifact is when the voided volume of urine is not completely captured by the collection funnel during the study, resulting in an underestimate of voided volume as well as flow rate. Particularly in men, the intravesical catheter should be carefully secured as to not interfere with the flow of urine from the meatus.

POSTSTUDY CONSIDERATIONS

The AUA best practice statement for urologic surgery antimicrobial prophylaxis recommends antibiotic prophylaxis for UDS only in patients with risk factors.[19] These risk factors include advanced age, anatomic anomalies of the urinary tract, poor nutritional status, smoking, chronic corticosteroid use, immunodeficiency, externalized catheters, colonized endogenous/exogenous material, distant coexistent infection, and prolonged hospitalization.

Interpretation of the UDS study should occur in real-time during the study and are discussed elsewhere in this issue.

SUMMARY

UDS is a collection of tests that when combined provides useful information with respect to urinary bladder filling/storage and emptying. The quality and results of the UDS study are operator-dependent and are only as good as the clinician who performs and interprets the study. In performing a quality UDS study, the clinician should formulate the UDS questions to be answered, properly design the study to answer those questions, be able to adapt the study as necessary, and recognize and correct artifacts that occur during the study.

REFERENCES

1. Schafer W, Abrams P, Liao L, et al. Good urodynamic practices: uroflowmetry, filling cystometry, and pressure-flow studies. Neurourol Urodyn 2002; 21(3):261–74.
2. Goode PS, Locher JL, Bryant RL, et al. Measurement of postvoid residual urine with portable transabdominal bladder ultrasound scanner and urethral catheterization. Int Urogynecol J Pelvic Floor Dysfunct 2000;11(5):296–300.
3. Yucel S, Kocak H, Sanli A, et al. How accurate is measuring postvoid residual volume by portable abdominal ultrasound equipment in peritoneal dialysis patient? Neurourol Urodyn 2005;24(4):358–61.
4. Rowan D, James ED, Kramer AE, et al. Urodynamic equipment: technical aspects. Produced by the International Continence Society working party on urodynamic equipment. J Med Eng Technol 1987;11(2):57–64.
5. Scarpero HM, Kaufman MR, Koski ME, et al. Urodynamics best practices. AUA Update Series 2009; 28:9.
6. Nitti VW. Urodynamic and video-urodynamic evaluation of the lower urinary tract. In: Wein A, Kavoussi LR, Novick AC, et al, editors. Campbell-Walsh urology. 10th edition. Philadelphia: Elsevier Saunders; 2012. p. 1847–70.
7. Rovner ES, Ginsberg DA. Radiology of urinary incontinence in the female. AUA Update Series 2002;21:22.
8. Winters JC, Dmochowski RR, Goldman HB, et al. Urodynamic studies in adults: AUA/SUFU guideline. J Urol 2012;188(Suppl 6):2464–72.
9. Scarpero HM, Padmanabhan P, Xue X, et al. Patient perception of videourodynamic testing: a questionnaire based study. J Urol 2005;173(2):555–9.
10. Gray M. Traces: making sense of urodynamics testing. Urol Nurs 2010;30(5):267–75.
11. Rovner ES, Wein AJ. Practical urodynamics: part I. AUA Update Series 2002;21:19.
12. Abrams P, Cardozo L, Fall M, et al. The standardisation of terminology in lower urinary tract function: report from the standardisation sub-committee of the International Continence Society. Urology 2003; 61(1):37–49.
13. McGuire EJ, Woodside JR, Borden TA, et al. Prognostic value of urodynamic testing in myelodysplastic patients. J Urol 1981;126(2):205–9.
14. van Waalwijk van Doorn ES, Remmers A, Janknegt RA. Conventional and extramural ambulatory urodynamic testing of the lower urinary tract in female volunteers. J Urol 1992;147(5):1319–25 [discussion: 1326].
15. Wyndaele JJ, De Wachter S. Cystometrical sensory data from a normal population: comparison of two groups of young healthy volunteers examined with 5 years interval. Eur Urol 2002;42(1):34–8.

16. Boschen MJ. Paruresis (psychogenic inhibition of micturition): cognitive behavioral formulation and treatment. Depress Anxiety 2008;25(11):903–12.

17. Gray M. Traces: making sense of urodynamics testing–part 10: evaluation of micturition via the voiding pressure-flow study. Urol Nurs 2012;32(2):71–8.

18. Gray M. Traces: making sense of urodynamics testing–part 3: electromyography of the pelvic floor muscles. Urol Nurs 2011;31(1):31–8.

19. Wolf JS Jr, Bennett CJ, Dmochowski RR, et al. Best practice policy statement on urologic surgery antimicrobial prophylaxis. J Urol 2008;179(4):1379–90.

Can Intrinsic Sphincter Deficiency be Diagnosed by Urodynamics?

 CrossMark

Lisa M. Parrillo, MD[a], Parvati Ramchandani, MD[a,b],
Ariana L. Smith, MD[c],*

KEYWORDS

- Stress urinary incontinence • Intrinsic sphincter deficiency • Urodynamics
- Valsalva leak point pressure • Maximal urethral closure pressure

KEY POINTS

- Stress urinary incontinence has historically been classified into 3 separate types based on anatomic configuration, urethral hypermobility, and urethral function; traditionally, these classifications helped direct surgical treatments.
- Urodynamics is a tool used to differentiate between types of stress incontinence. In spite of practice guidelines from the International Continence Society, not all aspects of urodynamic testing are standardized and the test can be challenging to perform.
- Intrinsic sphincter deficiency (ISD) is diagnosed by using urodynamics to measure Valsalva leak point pressure or maximal urethral closure pressures (MUCP), which can be difficult to interpret given natural variations in MUCP in both continent and incontinent women, and the potential different techniques that can be used during testing.
- Retropubic midurethral slings may have a higher success rate than transobturator midurethral slings in women with ISD.
- Being able to more accurately diagnose ISD before surgery may allow for the tailoring of surgical procedures to patients thereby improving success rates.

INTRODUCTION

Intrinsic sphincter deficiency (ISD) is a pathologic condition that can lead to female stress urinary incontinence (SUI), a condition that affects approximately 22% of women aged 45 to 64 years.[1] SUI is currently defined by the International Continence Society (ICS) as "the complaint of involuntary loss of urine on effort or physical exertion or on sneezing or coughing."[2] Clinically, one will observe leakage of urine per urethra provoked by synchronous activity that increases intra-abdominal pressure (ie, coughing, Valsalva). In women, the causes of SUI are multifactorial, but to some degree are attributable to urethral hypermobility, impaired sphincteric function, or a combination of the two. Defining the causes of SUI was believed to be helpful when counseling patients about the available surgical options and response to therapy, but as will be discussed later, this article is no longer as important, due to advances in the surgical techniques.

Disclosures: None.
[a] Division of Urology, Department of Surgery, Hospital of the University of Pennsylvania, 3400 Spruce Street, Philadelphia, PA 19104, USA; [b] Department of Radiology, Hospital of the University of Pennsylvania, 3400 Spruce Street, Philadelphia, PA 19104, USA; [c] Division of Urology, Department of Surgery, Perelman School of Medicine, 800 Walnut Street, Floor 19, Philadelphia, PA 19104, USA
* Corresponding author.
E-mail address: Ariana.smith@uphs.upenn.edu

HISTORY

In an effort to facilitate appropriate diagnosis and treatment, SUI was classified by Green in 1962 based on the anatomic configuration of the bladder and the urethra. Type I SUI was defined as the loss of a normal posterior urethrovesical angle and support of the bladder neck. On fluoroscopy, one would visualize a straightening of the posterior urethrovesical angle to greater than 180° with straining. Urethral pressure measured by urodynamics would show a maximal urethral closure pressure (MUCP) in the proximal urethra to be greater than 20 cm H_2O.[3] Women with Type II SUI demonstrated not only straightening of the posterior urethrovesical angle but also experienced hypermobility of the proximal urethra and bladder neck, which was seen as a shift down and back of greater than 3 cm (vs only 2–3 cm in those with Type I SUI) with straining. Again, the MUCP was measured greater than 20 cm H_2O. In both Type I and Type II SUI, a rise in intra-abdominal pressure is not equally distributed between the bladder and the posterior urethra once the urethra has descended out of its normal anatomic position. The increased pressure experienced by the bladder relative to the urethra produces a pressure differential and facilitates leakage.[4,5] In the 1970s, McGuire reported an additional cause of SUI, which has since been labeled Type III.[5] In these patients, there was no urethral hypermobility, but the bladder neck and proximal urethra did not function properly, which was thought to be associated with low closure pressures.[3] Type III SUI was also referred to as ISD and is associated with an MUCP less than 20 cm H_2O.[6,7]

Historically, the clinical categorization of SUI was considered an important factor in the determination of treatment, specifically which surgical intervention to use. Certain surgical interventions, like injection of urethral bulking agents, which are aimed at augmenting compression and increasing resistance of the mid- to proximal urethra, were found to improve symptoms in some women with Type III SUI, but still had higher failure rates in patients with both low Valsalva leak point pressures (less than 60 cm H_2O) and MUCPs (less than 20 cm H_2O).[8,9] Retropubic urethral suspension procedures, which are aimed at preventing mobility of the bladder neck and urethra, were found to be most effective in those with Type I or Type II SUI.[10] Mechanistically, these findings made conceptual sense and further supported the categorization of SUI. With the advent of the suburethral sling procedure, first placed at the bladder neck and more recently placed at the midurethra, the categorization of SUI has become less important as the sling has been deemed effective in all categories of SUI.[11] However, there is continued interest in predicting response to surgery as some evidence suggests slightly improved dry rates following a sling for women with urethral hypermobility versus those with ISD.[12]

USING URODYNAMICS TO EVALUATE SUI

When it is important for the clinician to establish the cause and type of SUI, urodynamics is commonly utilized. The goal of urodynamics in a patient presenting with SUI is to objectively measure, in a way that is quantifiable, the lower urinary tract function of each patient and to find a physiologic reason for their subjective symptoms. The 2002 ICS "Good Urodynamic Practices" report recommends first obtaining a clear history, including a voiding diary, and performing a thorough physical examination, which could include a cough stress test. The clinician may also want to obtain noninvasive urinary flow rate and postvoid residual urine volume measurement if indicated by the clinical scenario. However, if attempting to define the types of SUI, invasive urodynamics (filling cystometry, pressure flow) would be needed. Invasive urodynamics uses a pressure transducer in the bladder and the rectum (or vagina) along with electromyography, which is most commonly obtained by surface electrode patches on the anal sphincter, measures lower urinary tract function, and helps identify the pathology behind the lower urinary tract symptoms. Urodynamic measures include bladder capacity; bladder compliance; abdominal leak point pressure (ALPP) (which can be induced by Valsalva leak point pressure or cough [cough leak point pressure]); MUCP; and the presence of observations such as detrusor overactivity, bladder outlet obstruction, detrusor sphincter dyssynergia, and underactive detrusor contraction.[13]

To standardize measurements during urodynamics, the ICS recommends establishing a detrusor pressure of zero at the start of the study by equalizing the vesicle and abdominal pressure transducers.[13] For fluid-filled systems, a reference height is established at a height that is equal to that of the upper edge of the pubic symphysis (as opposed to air charged, which do not require this reference point). A dual lumen transurethral catheter is usually used to measure intravesical pressure and allow for simultaneous bladder filling. A rectal (or vaginal) catheter is used for the measurement of abdominal pressure. It is also recommended that the display include 3 measurement channels: a method of displaying and storing pressure data; the ability to accurately measure pressure from 0 to 250 cm H_2O, flow from 0 to 50 mL/s, and volume up to 1000 mL; and a standard scale for displaying data. All equipments should be appropriately and regularly calibrated. To help achieve accurate measurements, the ICS recommends assuring that resting values are appropriate, abdominal and intravesical pressures vary similarly with breath or movement, and that coughs are regularly used to be sure of equivalent abdominal and intravesical response. Finally, it is suggested that urodynamic testing should be repeated to confirm reproducibility of the results before initiating treatment.[14]

Even with these guidelines in place, urodynamic testing can be challenging. There are many additional factors that can be altered during testing. These alterations undoubtedly affect results and are without standardized guidelines from the ICS currently. These will be discussed in greater detail later with specific relation to ISD. Additionally, the reliability and reproducibility of urodynamics has been discussed by the ICS. During the evaluation of SUI, and specifically ISD, careful attention is paid to the values of ALPP and MUCP. There are no standard recommendations for positioning during urodynamics, and in a 2002 study out of UCLA, the effect of positioning on leak point pressure was evaluated. Thirty-seven patients with SUI and 4 with mixed incontinence underwent measurement of leak point pressures while in supine, semirecumbent, and standing positions. They found that leaking occurred with less intravesical pressure as the patient went from supine to standing position.[15]

It has been noted in the literature that there are differences in MUCP depending on the type of catheter used. In a 2008 prospective study by Zehnder, 64 women were randomized to undergo MUCP measurements first with either an air-charged catheter or a microtip catheter used. MUCP was then measured again with the other type of catheter. Mean MUCP was significantly higher with the use of an air-charged catheter, but the repeatability of measurements was stable for both catheters. Therefore, although the measurement of MUCP may be trusted to be reproducible for a given woman, it is challenging to establish reference ranges and compare data across studies without standardization of catheter type.[16]

USING URODYNAMICS TO DIAGNOSE ISD

ISD is believed to be due to deficiencies in the urethral and periurethral tissues that result in weakness of the sphincteric mechanism. These weaknesses can result from age, pregnancy, and childbirth; the development of a neurologic injury; or from previous surgical or radiation therapies. Clinically, urethral function is objectively measured by ALPP and MUCP. ALPP is defined by the ICS as the intravesical pressure at which urine leakage occurs due to increased abdominal pressure in the absence of a detrusor contraction. MUCP is the highest pressure, relative to bladder pressure, generated along the length of the urethra. The literature has suggested that both a low MUCP and ALPP be used to diagnose ISD,[17] and the cutoff values most commonly recommended are an ALPP less than 60 cm H_2O and a MUCP less that 20 cm.[18]

Part of the challenge with reliably diagnosing ISD with urodynamics is a lack of true consensus on how exactly the ALPP and MUCP are measured. McGuire initially described ISD as being a loss of tone that manifested itself as a low proximal urethral pressure. He advocated using fluoroscopy during urodynamics to appropriately position a catheter in the proximal urethra while measuring urethral pressures, as this was the "part of the urethra concerned with resistance to abdominal pressure as an expulsive force."[19] In the early 1990s, McGuire introduced a new urodynamic measure that he believed was better correlated with ISD, the ALPP.

McGuire's technique for testing ALPP is as follows: first the flow pressure of the system must be zeroed. Then, the bladder is filled at 60 mL/minute until the bladder contains approximately 200 to 250 mL of fluid. The patient is placed in an upright position, maintaining the transducer at the height of the pubic symphysis, and is asked to perform a slow, progressive Valsalva until leakage occurs. He recommends repeating the study several times to obtain an average abdominal pressure at the moment of leakage.[20]

As mentioned, a diagnosis of ISD is based on abnormal measurements of ALPP and MUCP. Hosker published a recent review of the literature focusing on the methods used to obtain these values clinically. From the studies he referenced it is clear that there is no set consensus on how exactly urodynamics is to be performed and interpreted when trying to identify ISD. Although it appears that the urologic community agrees that ALPP of 60 H_2O is a requirement for diagnosing ISD, there were different definitions for the cutoff for MUCP. Most studies used an MUCP of 20 cm H_2O, but some used 15 H_2O or 30 H_2O as their parameter for ISD.

Furthermore, the methodologies for measuring MUCP and ALPP varied significantly. They were measured with an empty bladder, with the bladder at capacity up to 500 mL, with150 mL in the bladder, with 250 mL in the bladder, and with a bladder volume between 200 and 300 mL. Patient positioning and catheter size were also not standardized. Measurements were obtained in the semirecumbent, standing, and upright sitting positions. Catheter sizes ranged from 7 to 10 French. Further divergence in technique could develop when considering the other components of urodynamic testing such as catheter withdrawal speed, viscosity of bladder fluid, rate of infusion, and the use of a Valsalva or a cough.[21]

Typically, MUCP is measured at rest, as opposed to ALPP, which is measured during an increase in intra-abdominal pressure, which simulates the real world scenario that leads to leakage. MUCP may reflect underlying deficiencies in the sphincteric function, but may miss deficiencies that are only notable during increases in intra-abdominal pressure. In addition to the association with degree of incontinence, MUCP has been found to correlate strongly with age, which suggests that the aging process weakens the intrinsic function of the urethra even in continent women. MUCP is also significantly decreased in women who have previously had anti-incontinence surgery.[22]

In **Table 1**, examples of normative urodynamic values of MUCP in women of various ages who are either continent or with stress incontinence are displayed. In both groups, MUCP is seen to decrease with age, but there is a wide range of MUCP in each age group, making it difficult to interpret and establish diagnoses. Of note, there are women who are continent and yet have MUCP less than 20 mm H_2O. Given this evidence that MUCP can vary with age and degree of incontinence, it complicates the interpretation of these data for diagnosis of ISD.

The natural decrease of MUCP with age is partially attributable to the loss of urethral tissue. For example, the density of circular smooth muscle is 25% to 50% higher in women in their 20s or 30s compared with that of women in their 70s of 80s.[24] Additionally, the number of striated muscle cells in the ventral wall of the urethra has also been noted to decrease over time, especially in the proximal urethra, just distal to the bladder neck. Over time, the mucosa also thins, connective tissue volume increases, and there is a loss of proteoglycans, all of which can lead to decreases in the urethral wall apposition.[25] Finally, MUCP has been noted to decrease steadily by about 15% with each decade of life.[26] On magnetic resonance imaging, it is possible to visualize the differences in urethral tissue between an elderly and a young woman. In **Figs. 1** and **2**, the urethra of an 81-year-old woman is compared with that of a 22-year-old woman. Although there is no reported methodology for measuring muscle thickness of the female urethra, it is easily discernable that there is a significant disparity in bulk.

Table 1 Maximal urethral closure pressure by age group			
	Women with ISD	Women with SUI	Continent Women
MUCP	<20 mm H_2O	Age group: mean (95% CI) 20–29: 70.35 (63.6–77.1) 30–39: 61.38 (59.3–63.5) 40–49: 54.44 (53.31–55.8) 50–59: 38.30 (47.0–49.6) 60–69: 39.42 (37.7–41.1) 70–79: 32.72 (30.5–34.9) 80+: 26.82 (21.52–32.1) MUCP <20 mm H_2O in 5.8% of women[22]	Age group: median (interquartile range) Premenopausal: 49 (37–72) Perimenopausal: 35 (29–46) Postmenopausal: 44 (33–43)[23] Age group: mean (95% CI) 20–29: 92.43 (88.1–96.8) 30–39: 80.71 (77.9–83.5) 40–49: 72.62 (70–3–74.9) 50–59: 60.84 (58.5–62.3) 60–69: 53.62 (50.5–56.8) 70–79: 46.81 (36.4–45.3) 80+: 39.60 (29.5–49.7) MUCP <20 mm H_2O in 1.4% of women[22]

Abbreviation: CI, confidence interval.

Data from Kapoor DS, Housami F, White P, et al. Maximum urethral closure pressure in women: normative data and evaluation as a diagnostic test. Int Urogynecol J 2012;23(11):1613–8; and Pfisterer M, Griffiths DJ, Rosenberg L, et al. Parameters of bladder function in pre-, peri-, and postmenopausal continent women without detrusor overactivity. Neurourol Urodyn 2007;26(3):356–61.

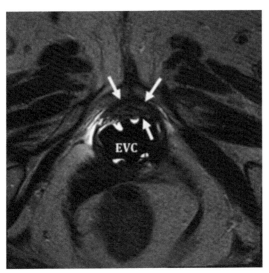

Fig. 1. Axial T2-weighted magnetic resonance imaging of urethra (*arrows*) in an 81-year-old woman, with urethral atrophy. EVC, endovaginal coil.

THE SURGICAL APPROACH TO ISD

Clinical experience has suggested that differentiating between Type I or Type II SUI and Type III SUI preoperatively may prove significant when counseling patients about the chances of relief from their symptoms after a procedure. Although the evidence is controversial, there are some studies that suggest that women with a diagnosis suggestive of ISD defined by a low ALPP or MUCP

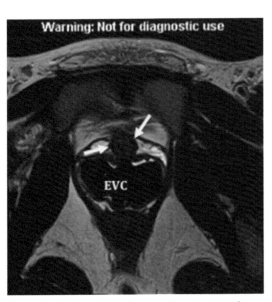

Fig. 2. Axial T2-weighted magnetic resonance imaging of urethra (*arrows*) in a 22-year-old woman with stress and urge incontinence, no significant urethral atrophy. EVC, endovaginal coil.

are more likely to fail midurethral sling procedures potentially because of poor coaptation or an immobile urethra.[27] In a review structured to determine the predictive value of urodynamics before an operative intervention for SUI, Kawasaki and colleagues[28] noted that with both retropubic and transobturator slings, there is a lower rate of post-operative cure in individuals with low MUCP, which was corroborated by the TOMUS trial, a randomized study comparing retropubic to transobturator midurethral slings. Although there was no apparent association between preoperative urodynamics and subjective failure, the lowest quartile of MUCP (45 cm H_2O) and ALPP (86 cm H_2O) before surgery were noted to increase the rate of objective failure significantly (P = .003 for both).[29]

One prospective studied look at women with SUI and ISD who were treated with a midurethral sling. These women were randomized to tension-free vaginal tape (TVT) or a transobturator midurethral tape (TOT) procedure. One hundred sixty-four women were randomized, 82 to each group, and there were no significant differences in demographics between the women. The diagnosis of ISD was established if the MUCP was less than 20 mm H_2O and the ALPP was less than 60 mm H_2O with the bladder filled to 500 cc or maximum capacity if less than 500 cc.[30] At 6-month follow-up, there was a notable distinction between the 2 groups: 13% in the TOT arm had already required additional surgery compared with 0% of the women with a TVT. At 3 years, the disparity between the 2 groups was still evident with 18.3% of the TOT women versus 1.2% of the TVT women undergoing another surgical procedure to correct SUI. The authors speculate that this difference may be secondary to a difference in sling axis or perhaps unintentional increased sling tension during surgery with placement of TVT. Regardless, these data seem to indicate that if a clinician is able to diagnose a woman with ISD before surgery, choosing to perform a TVT may lead to higher continence success rates.[31]

CAN ISD BE DIAGNOSED BY URODYNAMICS

When faced with answering the question of whether or not ISD can be diagnosed by urodynamics, the answer is more complicated than a simple yes or no. As a community, urologists and urogynecologists need to establish universal definitions and standards so the women whose SUI is attributable to ISD can be better diagnosed. There is fairly good consensus that ISD is present with an ALPP less than 60 mm H_2O and an MUCP of less than 20 mm H_2O, but discrepancies in the literature do exist, most commonly regarding the MUCP. Settling those discrepancies will be challenging and will likely require additional studies to assess the technical components of ALPP and MUCP measurements, as well as the reliability of particular cutoffs in predicting ISD.

Urodynamics, as a diagnostic test, can certainly be valuable, but it is difficult to compare results across practices and establish treatment guidelines when methodologies vary widely. Good urodynamics practice guidelines have established several important standards; however, clarity on measurement of ALPP and MUCP is needed. It would be advantageous to establish recommendations for measurement to allow comparisons across practices and research studies with respect to severity of SUI disease and response to therapy. In the meantime, consistent methodology in one's personal practice may be helpful to understanding the differences among patients. One important consideration in the development of standard techniques for the measurement of ALPP and MUCP is patient positioning. It would be reasonable to evaluate those patients who are thought to have ISD in a situation that would cause them to have the most leakage, which is standing up. This situation however may lead to recruitment of accessory pelvic floor muscles that alter pressure measurements compared with the seated or supine position. It is also important to standardize bladder volume at the time of pressure measurement because capacity will likely influence the chance of leakage and pressure dynamics.

One might question why the diagnosis of ISD even matters if the contemporary treatment plan is the same, with the placement of a midurethral sling, regardless of the type of SUI present. However, it is known that slings fail and it is thought that they fail more commonly in patients with ISD. The exact reason for these failures and the exact mechanism by which a sling improves leakage in the setting of ISD remain unknown. The authors believe assessment for ISD can be beneficial in preoperative patient counseling: women with ISD who may be anticipated to fail slings can have their expectations appropriately tempered by preoperative counseling.

Additionally, more reliable and better-defined diagnoses of ISD may impact future treatment development. As surgical techniques evolve, being able to precisely measure urethral deficiency with quantitative, comparable values could lead to more directed care and potentially better outcomes. Specifically, populations for which a specific treatment such as TVT or TOT may be more efficacious may be defined with further research. Tailoring the surgical procedure to quantitative

preoperative data or measuring MUCP during midurethral sling placement may have the ability to improve surgical success.

It is clear that although urodynamics provides important information pertaining to ISD, this information is not comparable across sites because acquisition techniques have not been standardized. Further studies in patients with ISD using standardized urodynamic methodologies and interpretations may allow for better understanding of the condition as well as more realistic preoperative planning and improved outcomes for women who are plagued by SUI.

REFERENCES

1. Shamliyan T, Wyman J, Bliss DZ, et al. Prevention of urinary and fecal incontinence in adults. Evid Rep Technol Assess (Full Rep) 2007;161:1–379.
2. Haylen BT, Freeman RM, Lee J, et al. An International Urogynecological Association (IUGA)/International Continence Society (ICS) joint report on the terminology for female pelvic floor dysfunction. Int Urogynecol J 2010;21(1):5–26.
3. McGuire EJ, Lytton B, Kohor EI, et al. The value of urodynamic testing in stress urinary incontinence. J Urol 1980;124(2):256–8.
4. Green T. Vaginal repair. In: Stanton SL, Tanagho EA, editors. Surgery of female incontinence. New York: Springer-Verlag; 1980. p. 31–46.
5. McGuire EJ, Lytton B, Pepe V, et al. Stress urinary incontinence. Obstet Gynecol 1976;47(3):255–64.
6. Arriola PR, Dalenz VS, Schanz JP. Study of female urinary incontinence with single channel urodynamics: comparison of the symptoms on admission. Analysis of 590 females. Neurological and urodynamic urology. Arch Esp Urol 2009;62(2):115–21 [in Spanish].
7. Wein A, Barrett D. Voiding function and dysfunction: a logical and practical approach. Chicago: Year Book Medical Publishing; 1988. p. 287–8.
8. Sanchez-Ortiz RF, Broderick GA, Chaikin DC, et al. Collagen injection therapy for post-radical retropubic prostatectomy incontinence: role of Valsalva leak point pressure. J Urol 1997;158(6):2132–6.
9. Gorton E, Stanton S, Monga A, et al. Periurethral collagen injection: a long-term follow-up study. BJU Int 1999;84:966–71.
10. Green TH Jr. The problem of urinary stress incontinence in the female: an appraisal of its current status. Obstet Gynecol Surv 1968;23(7):603–34.
11. Chaikin DC, Rosenthal J, Blaivas J. Pubovaginal fascial sling for all types of stress urinary incontinence: long-term analysis. J Urol 1998;160(4):1312–6.
12. Minaglia S, Urwitz-Lane R, Wong M, et al. Effectiveness of transobturator tape in women with

decreased urethral mobility. J Reprod Med 2009; 54(1):15–9.

13. Rosier P, Kuo HC, De Gennaro M, et al. Urodynamic testing. In: Abrams P, Cardozo L, Khoury S, et al, editors. Incontinence: 5th International consultation on incontinence. 2013. p. 429–506.

14. Schäfer W, Abrams P, Liao L, et al. Good urodynamic practices: uroflowmetry, filling cystometry, and pressure-flow studies. Neurourol Urodyn 2002; 21(3):261–74.

15. Nguyen JK, Gunn GC, Bhatia NN. The effect of patient position on leak-point pressure measurements in women with genuine stress incontinence. Int Urogynecol J 2002;13(1):9–14.

16. Zehnder P, Roth B, Burkhard FC, et al. Air charged and microtip catheters cannot be used interchangeably for urethral pressure measurement: a prospective, single-blind, randomized trial. J Urol 2008;180(3):1013–7.

17. Bump RC, Coates KW, Cundiff GW, et al. Diagnosing intrinsic sphincteric deficiency: comparing urethral closure pressure, urethral axis, and Valsalva leak point pressures. Am J Obstet Gynecol 1997;177(2):303–10.

18. Swift S. Intrinsic sphincter deficiency: what is it and does it matter anymore? Int Urogynecol J 2012; 24(2):1–2.

19. McGuire EJ. Urodynamic evaluation of stress incontinence. Urol Clin North Am 1995;22(3):551.

20. McGuire EJ, Cespedes RD, O'Connell HE. Leak-point pressures. Urol Clin North Am 1996;23:253–62.

21. Hosker G. Is it possible to diagnose intrinsic sphincter deficiency in women? Curr Opin Urol 2009;19(4):342–6.

22. Kapoor DS, Housami F, White P, et al. Maximum urethral closure pressure in women: normative data and evaluation as a diagnostic test. Int Urogynecol J 2012;23(11):1613–8.

23. Pfisterer M, Griffiths DJ, Rosenberg L, et al. Parameters of bladder function in pre-, peri-, and postmenopausal continent women without detrusor overactivity. Neurourol Urodyn 2007;26(3):356–61.

24. Clobes A, DeLancey JO, Morgan DM. Urethral circular smooth muscle in young and old women. Am J Obstet Gynecol 2008;198(5):587.e1–5.

25. Verelst M, Maltau JM, Ørbo A. Computerised morphometric study of the paraurethral tissue in young and elderly women. Neurourol Urodyn 2002; 21(6):529–33.

26. DeLancey JO. Why do women have stress urinary incontinence? Neurourol Urodyn 2010;29(Suppl 1): S13–7.

27. Stav K, Dwyer PL, Rosamilia A, et al. Risk factors of treatment failure of midurethral sling procedures for women with urinary stress incontinence. Int Urogynecol J 2010;21(2):149–55.

28. Kawasaki A, Wu JM, Amundsen CL, et al. Do urodynamic parameters predict persistent postoperative stress incontinence after midurethral sling? A systematic review. Int Urogynecol J 2012;23(7): 813–22.

29. Nager CW, Sirls L, Litman HJ, et al. Baseline urodynamic predictors of treatment failure 1 year after mid urethral sling surgery. J Urol 2011; 186(2):597–603.

30. Schierlitz L, Dwyer PL, Rosamilia A, et al. Effectiveness of tension-free vaginal tape compared with transobturator tape in women with stress urinary incontinence and intrinsic sphincter deficiency: a randomized controlled trial. Obstet Gynecol 2008; 112(6):1253–61.

31. Schierlitz L, Dwyer PL, Rosamilia A, et al. Three-year follow-up of tension-free vaginal tape compared with transobturator tape in women with stress urinary incontinence and intrinsic sphincter deficiency. Obstet Gynecol 2012;119(2 Pt 1):321–7.

Videourodynamics
Indications and Technique

Brian K. Marks, MD[a],*, Howard B. Goldman, MD[b]

KEYWORDS

- Videourodynamics • Fluoroscopy • Neurogenic bladder • Bladder outlet obstruction
- Primary bladder neck obstruction • Guidelines

KEY POINTS

- Videourodynamics (VUDS) combines a fluoroscopic voiding cystourethrogram with multichannel urodynamics, allowing anatomic and functional assessment of the bladder and outlet.
- There is a relative paucity of guidelines and literature surrounding the specific indications and techniques for VUDS.
- A thorough patient assessment is paramount in developing a differential diagnosis and identifying urodynamic questions to be answered.
- VUDS should be considered in patients with neurologic findings or diseases as well as those with obstructed voiding, congenital genitourinary anomalies, or a history of genitourinary reconstruction.
- Appropriate use of fluoroscopy is important in reducing any added cost and risk of ionizing radiation to patients and clinical staff.

INTRODUCTION

Diagnosing patients with multiple lower urinary tract symptoms and confounding comorbidities may require further assessment with advanced diagnostic testing, such as urodynamics. Standard multichannel urodynamics most often includes a filling cystometrogram and a pressure flow study during micturition. These 2 components are often the only obligatory tests required to determine a diagnosis; however, key pathognomonic findings may be overlooked in certain patient populations. Further delineation may be required, and the use of concomitant radiologic imaging during the study provides additional data to hone the differential diagnosis. Fluoroscopic imaging has been the modality of choice as an adjunct to traditional urodynamics.

Combining fluoroscopic voiding cystourethrogram with pressure flow urodynamics to evaluate lower urinary tract function dates back to the 1950s, was further developed through the 1970s, and was not widely used clinically until the 1980s.[1–3] The original set-up used analog portable fluoroscopy (C-arm) and signal processing to combine the oscilloscope tracing from the pressure transducer with the live fluoroscopic images.[2,3] This allowed simultaneous recording on a magnetic tape for cine image viewing, hence, the coined term, *VUDS*.

Improvements in portable computing and digital signal processing paved the way for modern-day VUDS (also referred to as fluoro-urodynamics). Imaging input (video) is channeled into a computer terminal with software chronologically integrating the digital image with the cystometrogram and pressure flow tracings. Advancements in imaging technology paralleled the changes in computing, and digital imaging detectors led to fully integrated

Disclosures: None.
[a] Center for Urologic Care, Concord Hospital, 246 Pleasant Street, Suite G2, Concord, NH 03301, USA;
[b] Glickman Urological and Kidney Institute, Cleveland Clinic, 9500 Euclid Avenue, Q10-1, Cleveland, OH 44195, USA
* Corresponding author.
E-mail address: bmarks@crhc.org

digital fluoroscopy. This has allowed easier combination of the 2 technologies and facilitates review of imaging on specialized medical image viewing software with improved resolution and tools to optimize image analysis.

VUDS provides additional information compared with standard urodynamics; however, use of this specialized test should be limited to patients in whom this information adds value. There is increased cost and risk associated with radiologic imaging and clinicians should consider the usefulness of adding fluoroscopy as part of a patient's evaluation.

INDICATIONS

Fluoroscopy as an adjunct to standard urodynamics should be considered in those patients whose diagnosis is aided by including this modality. Specialty societies have developed guidelines for standardizing terminology and technique as well as clinical guidelines for use of urodynamics.[4,5] These guidelines are a consortium of expert panel opinion and literature review. A majority of recommendations apply to standard urodynamics and there is a paucity of guidelines and literature surrounding the specific indications and techniques for VUDS. Information in this article is derived from guidelines and available literature; however, much of the described principles and techniques follow expert opinion and the authors' standard practice.

Determining the patient populations that may benefit from VUDS requires clinicians to develop a differential diagnosis of underlying conditions that may contribute to a patient's urinary tract symptoms. This begins with a detailed history and physical examination. The history should include comorbid conditions and querying for any neurologic dysfunction as well as a family history of neurologic and congenital conditions. Knowledge of congenital anomalies and previous surgeries, in particular those involving the genitourinary or neurologic system, aids in patient selection. During examination, clinicians should evaluate for any signs of neurologic disease by assessing perineal sensation, pelvic muscle, and sphincter tone; testing the bulbocavernosus reflex; and identifying peripheral neuropathy or abnormalities of the vertebral column. In men, prostate size should be noted and the external urethral anatomy examined. In women, the examination includes evaluation of urethral mobility, incontinence, periurethral anatomy, and pelvic organ prolapse. Thorough assessment guides clinicians in formulating the diagnostic questions necessary to select the relevant urodynamic components.

Patients who may benefit from VUDS include those with neurologic findings or a history of neurologic disease, a history of congenital genitourinary anomalies, symptoms of obstructive voiding (often excluding straight forward benign prostate enlargement [BPE] symptoms), a history of pelvic irradiation, and a past history of surgical reconstruction. Current guidelines jointly published by the American Urological Association (AUA) and the Society of Urodynamics, Female Pelvic Medicine and Urogenital Reconstruction (SUFU) make only 2 recommendations regarding the use of VUDS.[5] These include recommending that clinicians may use fluoroscopy at the time of urodynamics in patients with relevant neurologic disease or those with an elevated postvoid residual or urinary symptoms and a neurologic condition that may contribute (guideline statement 12).[5] The other recommended condition is in patients with outlet obstruction to localize the level of obstruction, particularly in those thought to have primary bladder outlet obstruction (PBNO) (guideline statement 19).[5]

The use of fluoroscopy during urodynamics can aid in further evaluation of

- Vesicoureteral reflux (VUR)
- Anatomic variations of the bladder, including trabeculations, saccules or diverticula, and filling defects
- Voiding dynamics in women with a cystocele or pelvic organ prolapse
- Bladder neck function and coordination during micturition
- Urethral pathology, such as strictures or diverticula
- Detrusor–external sphincter dyssynergia (DESD) (in conjunction with sphincter electromyography [EMG])
- Dysfunctional voiding/pelvic floor dysfunction
- Urinary fistulas
- Urinary incontinence

Neurogenic Bladder

VUDS is often useful in the evaluation of patients with suspected neurogenic lower urinary tract dysfunction (NLUTD). Clinical diagnoses include spinal cord injury; spina bifida or spinal dysraphism; Parkinson disease; Shy-Drager syndrome (multiple system atrophy [MSA]); demyelinating disorders, such as multiple sclerosis; Devic disease; and transverse myelitis and, in some cases, diabetic neuropathy and following a cerebrovascular incident. This list is not all inclusive and clinical acumen is needed to determine other signs, symptoms, and underlying pathology that may lead to neurologic dysfunction.

Key pathognomonic findings in NLUTD that are better evaluated with VUDS include VUR, which may indicate poor bladder compliance, and identifying improper coordination between detrusor contraction and sphincter relaxation. Either of these findings typically represents neurogenic bladder, and, if a neurologic disease is not known, these findings should prompt exclusion of a potential neurologic disease. **Fig. 1** demonstrates 2 cases of bilateral VUR that occurs with bladder filling. In both cases, detrusor pressure remained normal and the only indication of bladder compliance changes was the identification of reflux. DESD occurs with lesions above the reflex pathways within the sacral spinal cord. With patch electrodes, the EMG tracing is not always diagnostic due to noise, and fluoroscopic findings may be the only evidence to suggest this condition (**Fig. 2**). Assessment of bladder contour may provide additional insight toward the underlying pathology. For example, trabeculations, multiple diverticula, or a Christmas tree appearance indicates obstruction, possibly related to neurogenic dysfunction, in those with a known neurologic condition.

Definite delineation between the lower urinary tract findings in MSA versus Parkinson disease requires concomitant fluoroscopic imaging to study bladder neck function. Multiple system atrophy demonstrates an open bladder neck during initial filling on fluoroscopy.[6] During micturition, patients with MSA have an open bladder neck with neurogenic sphincter motor potentials on EMG and fluoroscopic evidence of DESD, features rarely found in Parkinson disease.[6] Without multichannel VUDS with EMG, distinguishing the urologic manifestations of these 2 diseases is not possible.

Obstructed Voiding

Symptoms of obstructed voiding may be related to anatomic or functional outlet obstruction. Not all symptoms carry a straightforward clinical diagnosis on presentation and further assessment with urodynamics may be useful. Traditional multichannel urodynamics identify bladder outlet obstruction, such as that found in BPE; however, certain patients may have more than one potential source of obstruction. Assessment of patients with a past history of genitourinary surgery involving the outlet (male outlet or urethral surgeries, suburethral sling, female pelvic organ prolapse reconstruction, or urethral diverticulectomy) may be improved via the images obtained during the voiding phase of VUDS.

Concomitant fluoroscopic imaging can help localize the level of obstruction during pressure flow studies. The presence of a prominent prostatic median lobe may be identified in men with prostatic enlargement. Identifying a large bladder diverticulum may reveal voiding dynamics indicative of a pressure sink, suggesting outlet obstruction in those where the pressure tracing itself is not conclusive (**Fig. 3**). The severity of a cystocele may be more obvious during micturition and visualizing the dynamic mobility may identify urethral kinking and retention of urine in the displaced portion of the bladder (**Fig. 4**).[7,8] These findings may explain symptoms of obstruction in such women in the absence of other pathologies that create bladder outlet obstruction.

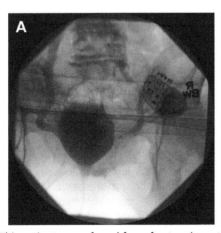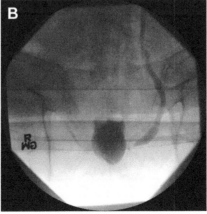

Fig. 1. (*A*) This patient was referred for refractory incontinence despite multiple treatment modalities, including sacral neuromodulation. Traditional urodynamics would not have identified the VUR and poor bladder compliance as the cause of her symptoms. (*B*) This patient with a past spinal cord injury demonstrates bilateral VUR early in bladder filling despite a normal detrusor pressure. Again, her compliance changes would not have been known without VUDS.

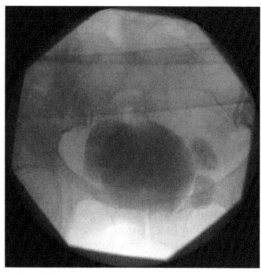

Fig. 3. In this woman with PBNO, measurable detrusor pressure remains low during micturition and the pressure is instead transmitted into the bladder diverticulum, visualized on the fluoroscopic images.

In women with obstructed voiding after anti-incontinence surgery, the necessity of urodynamics has been debated. In those with obstructive symptoms and evidence of retention or elevated PVR immediately after and temporally related to surgery, urodynamics is not likely needed.[9] In those with primary storage symptoms, urodynamics may be helpful, but clinical outcomes after surgical correction (sling incision or urethrolysis) are reported to be no different in those with or without diagnostic urodynamics.[9] VUDS may be useful in identifying the anatomic point of obstruction, as shown in **Fig. 5**. The study will be most useful in women whose clinical history is less clear and may be more useful in ruling out other causes of obstructing symptoms, such as dysfunctional voiding or primary bladder neck obstruction.

In men and women, VUDS facilitates analysis of coordinated micturition. This may be especially important in younger men and women without clinically apparent causes of obstructive voiding, such as BPE, prolapse, or prior surgery. Specifically, the function of the bladder neck, the external sphincter, and the pelvic floor can be studied with fluoroscopy. This may be useful in patients with primary bladder neck outlet obstruction and pelvic floor dysfunction. VUDS evaluation is the only diagnostic tool that can document pressure flow parameters and localize functional obstruction of the bladder neck.[5] Defining dysfunctional voiding as intermittent or fluctuating flow secondary to contractions of the periurethral striated muscle in a neurologically normal woman and PBNO as failure of bladder neck opening

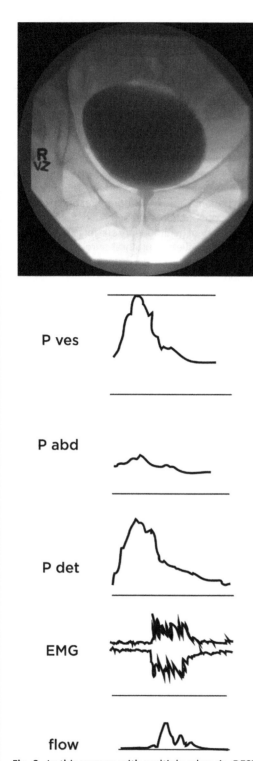

Fig. 2. In this woman with multiple sclerosis, DESD is evident with fluoroscopy during micturition. In this case, note both failure of relaxation of the bladder neck and the external sphincter. The pressure flow and EMG tracing reflect obstruction with increased sphincter motor potentials. P abd, abdominal pressure; P ves, vesical pressure; P det, detrusor pressure.

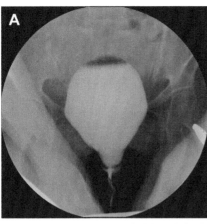
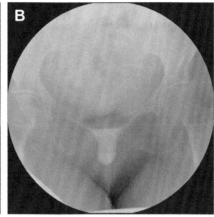

Fig. 4. In this woman with a stage II cystocele, residual urine is retained in the dependent portion of the bladder after voiding. (*A*) Voiding phase. (*B*) Post void residual.

resulting in obstructed voiding, one study found that EMG analysis alone would have incorrectly diagnosed 14% of women with PBNO as having dysfunctional voiding.[10] EMG activity alone, especially patch electrodes, has a high rate of inaccuracy in detecting quiescence during micturition, and using concomitant fluoroscopy increases the sensitivity and specificity of diagnosing dysfunctional voiding to 79% and 85%, respectively.[10] Note the difference between bladder neck function in a normal void compared with PBNO as presented in the VUDS images (**Fig. 6**).

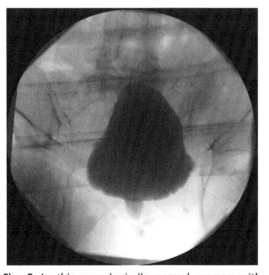

Fig. 5. In this neurologically normal woman with obstructive voiding symptoms and a remote history of a synthetic midurethral sling, the point of obstruction is identifiable along the urethra during voiding. Note funneling of the bladder neck with a very prominent urethra full of contrast and tapering to the point of obstruction.

Congenital Genitourinary Anomalies or History of Reconstruction

Clinicians should consider the use of VUDS in patients with a past history of congenital genitourinary anomalies or surgical correction of such anomalies. Important conditions include a childhood history of ureteropelvic junction obstruction, VUR, ectopic ureter, posterior urethral valves, or prune-belly syndrome, many of which are associated with other lower urinary tract pathology. Findings implicating these conditions include recurrent lower urinary tract infections or pyelonephritis, incomplete bladder emptying, and incontinence as well as the presence of hydronephrosis. Imaging can identify persistent or recurrent VUR as well as the presence of bladder trabeculations or diverticula. A paucity of outcomes data exists in evaluating the benefits of VUDS in the adult population with a past history of congenital anomalies and clinical judgment must be used as to whether added benefit is expected.

VUDS TECHNIQUE

Guidelines have been published for urodyamics by the International Continence Society (ICS) and the AUA/SUFU. The basic guidelines address indications and standardization of terminology.[4,5] The ICS guidelines set requirements for minimum equipment capabilities, required parameters to be measured, and calibration standards.[4] These guidelines ensure versatility in performing and reading urodynamic studies. The ICS guideline mentions that quantitative analysis may be supplemented by imaging (fluoroscopy or VUDS) and the AUA guidelines include 2 indications (discussed previously), but specific information regarding the technique and optimizing outcomes is not

A

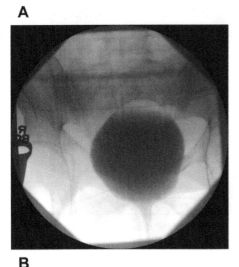

B

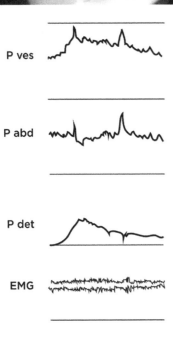

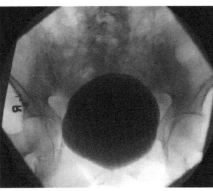

discussed.[4,5] In part, this is secondary to the paucity of outcomes-driven data available.

In general, the urodynamics set-up is similar to standard multichannel urodynamics but includes additional capabilities of integrating imaging (most commonly fluoroscopy) with the urodynamics tracings. VUDS essentially combines a voiding cystourethrogram with the cystometrogram and pressure flow tracings in standard multichannel urodynamics.

The components of VUDS typically include

- Initial noninvasive free flow
- Cystometrogram
- Pressure flow measurements
- EMG potentials representative of the external urinary sphincter
- Fluoroscopy for the voiding cystourethrogram

Equipment

Multichannel urodynamics

The mainstay equipment remains similar for that needed in traditional urodynamics. A multichannel urodynamics machine is required. The terminal should have an additional input for the video signal from fluoroscopy. Standards should meet those set forth by the ICS. Software integrates the image signal to the corresponding time point along the urodynamics tracing.

Fluoroscopy

Fluoroscopy is the most widely used imaging modality in urodynamics. A typical set-up uses a freestanding C-arm fluoroscopy machine, but an integrated fluoroscopy table may be used. Modern fluoroscopy machines produce a digital image.[11] The potential benefit of these devices is the lower radiation dose necessary for image acquisition secondary to digital detectors and automated control logic that reduces exposure.[11] Live image output is typically transmitted from the fluoroscopy unit to the terminal via coaxial cable.

A facility operating radiologic equipment is often subject to safety requirements set forth by regulatory bodies. These vary depending on geographic location but typically include standards for the facility or room in which the device is operated and the credentialing of the operating technician. Ionizing radiation has inherent risk and guidelines

---

Fig. 6. (A) Normal micturition demonstrates funneling of the bladder neck. (B) This VUDS study demonstrates failure of the bladder neck to funnel during voiding along with quiescence of the EMG on the urodynamics tracing, suggestive of PBNO. P abd, abdominal pressure; P ves, vesical pressure; P det, detrusor pressure.

must be followed to ensure the safety of patients and staff.

Contrast

Soluble iodized contrast medium replaces sterile water as the infusion medium for visualization with fluoroscopic imaging. Common formulations are iothalamate meglumine and diatrizoate meglumine, in low concentrations (17.2% and 18%, respectively) making the viscosity closer to that of water.[12] These agents are intended for extravascular use only. The solutions are often more viscous than water and the urodynamics equipment must be specifically calibrated to account for the viscosity of the chosen contrast media. This ensures the accuracy of the infused volume, voided volume, and flow rate. Provider practices vary and these agents are often further diluted with sterile water or saline. Few data exist evaluating the clinical outcomes when using diluted contrast. A single study evaluating the interpretability of fluoroscopic images during urodynamics, using 250 mL of contrast followed by saline, however, demonstrated no difference in interpretability.[13]

Specialized fluoroscopy table

Acquiring images during a study may be challenging. Reproducing symptoms is key in generating meaningful results and recreating the normal ergonomics of micturition is important in reproduction of symptoms. Using fluoroscopy requires positioning for image acquisition with the C-arm. In men, who stand upright to void, positioning of the C-arm to image the pelvis while voiding may be simple. In those patients who sit to void, specialized fluoroscopy tables may be helpful. These tables permit transmission of the radiograph and allow patients to position themselves in a more natural stance. They often have a cutout, allowing urine to easily direct into the uroflowmetry in a seated position.

Set-Up and Technique

Multichannel urodynamics are set up according to ICS guidelines.[4] The bladder is catheterized for the postvoid volume, ensuring an empty bladder before starting urodynamics. Similar to traditional pressure flow recordings, the pressure transducers are zeroed to atmosphere at the level of the pubic symphysis. Typically, a 7-French duel-lumen filling and recording catheter is inserted into the bladder to obtain intravesical pressure. A single-lumen rectal catheter is inserted to estimate abdominal pressure. The difference between these pressures estimates the pressure generated by the detrusor muscle. EMG electrodes are adhered to the region around the anal sphincter if indicated.

Filling cystometry is performed according to ICS guidelines, and the infusion pump is calibrated to account for the viscosity of the intravesical contrast agent. When switching between contrast media and water, the urodynamics technician must verify that the proper calibration setting is selected on the terminal.

Patients are typically placed in either a natural seated position or standing position using a specialized fluoroscopy table. Sequential fluoroscopic images are obtained, typically in an anterior-posterior view focusing on the pelvis. Urodynamicists may include a lateral or oblique view to better visualize the sagittal plane of the urethra as well as any mobility of the bladder, such as in pelvic organ prolapse. It is important to include the anatomic location of the urethra within the field of view for proper assessment during micturition. The number and timing of images typically vary based on local protocol. Few data exist on optimized image sequence, and guidelines do not address any recommended protocol. In general, a prefilling or scout image should be acquired as a baseline. The next image in sequence should follow early in filling to ensure that the bladder is filling properly, that contrast can be visualized, and to rule out VUR, posterior urethral anomalies, or extravasation. Voiding images are obtained to assess the bladder neck and urethra during micturition. A postvoid film may identify residual contrast that pools in a bladder diverticulum or cystocele (see **Fig. 4**)

Data have been published regarding safety of image acquisition. Newer digital fluoroscopy uses less radiation than older counterparts; however, total dose accumulation remains a concern, not only for patients but also for operators. Effort is being made to reduce the dose of ionizing radiation in medical imaging. Reduction of total accumulated dose is achieved if a total of only 4 to 5 images is acquired.[14] Timing of these images according to one center's protocol includes 1 image obtained at baseline (scout), 1 during filling, 1 image during a Valsalva, 1 image during voiding, and 1 repeated image during voiding if the catheter needs to be removed.[14] This protocol was able to reduce patients' dose of ionizing radiation by a factor of 3 without altering the interpretation of the urodynamic studies.[14] This is just a recommendation and if the particular question to be answered requires more images or continuous fluoroscopy, that is appropriate.

The key use for fluoroscopic imaging during urodynamics is to assess for functional storage problems and functional or anatomic voiding problems. During filling, urodynamacist must be diligent to identify VUR, a possible indicator for poor bladder compliance, as well as evidence of a bladder diverticulum, which may act as a pressure sink and mask evidence of outlet obstruction (see **Figs. 1** and **3**). In men with prostate enlargement, an intravesical median lobe may be readily apparent. The general urodynamics protocol for assessing incontinence includes generation of intravesical pressure with Valsalva or cough, and use of fluoroscopy may help identify incontinence as well as bladder mobility.[4] A cystocele that was present on physical examination may look more prominent on imaging and is best viewed in both anterior-posterior and lateral or oblique views. If obstruction is considered on the pressure flow tracing and a significant cystocele is noted, repeating the pressure flow with cystocele reduction may be considered to determine if outlet resistance was increased by the descending pelvic organ prolapse and to identify any occult incontinence (stress incontinence on prolapse reduction or latent stress incontinence).[7,8,15]

During micturition, imaging may identify VUR that occurs during voiding that was not present during fill, suggesting a pop-off mechanism at higher voiding pressures. The bladder neck should demonstrate relaxation or funneling during micturition, typically easier to identify in women because the prostate shadow often obscures this area in men (see **Fig. 6**A). The urethra should additionally be visualized to identify any narrowing of the urine stream or cutoff points that may suggest either anatomic obstruction from a stricture or prior reconstruction (such as a suburethral sling) versus functional obstruction from improperly coordinated relaxation of the external urinary sphincter or levator musculature. In cases of patients with a known neurologic condition, this likely represents DESD and can be compared with EMG data. Often, the patch electrodes from the EMG produce a poor tracing, and the fluoroscopic image may be the only data available to correlate with a patient's symptoms.

Additional information may be derived from the fluoroscopic images, not specific to the dynamics of voiding, but those that may not be readily evident in a history and physical examination. The observer should note any filling defects that may require further assessment with cystoscopy or advanced imaging. Filling defects may represent bladder tumors, urolithiasis, foreign body, or even sediment in the urine (often visualized as layering). Although rarely identified on voiding cystourethrogram imaging during VUDS, a urethral diverticulum may be evident lateral to or superimposed along the urethra and may be the cause of incontinence or obstructive voiding symptoms.

Limitations

Although a useful diagnostic test in the properly selected population, there are limitations to the capabilities of VUDS. As with traditional urodynamics, there is a subset of patients who are not able to micturate during the study. The cause is likely multifactorial, but the proportion of nonvoiders increases for VUDS.[8,15,16] Possible contributing factors include the presence of a urethral catheter, physical and psychological discomfort from the procedure, the unusual voiding environment that does not imitate the usual socially acceptable conditions for micturition, and even the voiding position required for the study, which often does not imitate the natural voiding posture patients assume in their own bathroom. Specifically with VUDS, the micturition position is less natural secondary to the need for a fluoroscopy table and the placement of the C-arm around a patient's pelvis. Another significant factor is probably the number of additional persons in the urodynamics suite during VUDS, often including a radiology technician, an operator (registered nurse, midlevel provider, or technician), and clinician.

SUMMARY

Appropriate and judicious use of VUDS lends to improved diagnostic acumen in well-selected patient populations. Paramount to obtaining useful data is proper patient selection, accomplished with a careful initial assessment focusing on symptoms, medical comorbidities, and past medical or surgical interventions. Guidelines specifically addressing selection between standard urodynamics versus the addition of fluoroscopic imaging are limited and outcomes data regarding technique are sparse. Clinicians must be mindful of the potential added cost, safety concerns, and limitations when considering the best study to further delineate a definitive diagnosis.

REFERENCES

1. Bates CP, Corney CE. Synchronous cine-pressure-flow cystography: a method of routine urodynamic investigation. Br J Radiol 1971;44(517):44–50.
2. Manoliu RA, Grimbergen HA, Ouwerkerk TJ, et al. Combined dynamic studies of the bladder and urethra. Report of a method. Eur Urol 1979;5(6):337–42.
3. Whiteside G, Bates P. Synchronous video pressure-flow cystourethrography. Urol Clin North Am 1979;6(1):93–102.
4. Schafer W, Abrams P, Liao L, et al. Good urodynamic practices: uroflowmetry, filling cystometry,

and pressure-flow studies. Neurourol Urodyn 2002; 21(3):261–74.

5. Winters JC, Dmochowski RR, Goldman HB, et al. Urodynamic studies in adults: AUA/SUFU guideline. J Urol 2012;188(Suppl 6):2464–72.

6. Sakakibara R, Hattori T, Uchiyama T, et al. Video-urodynamic and sphincter motor unit potential analyses in Parkinson's disease and multiple system atrophy. J Neurol Neurosurg Psychiatr 2001;71(5): 600–6.

7. Chaikin DC, Groutz A, Blaivas JG. Predicting the need for anti-incontinence surgery in continent women undergoing repair of severe urogenital prolapse. J Urol 2000;163(2):531–4.

8. Rovner ES, Banner MP, Ramchandani P, et al. Clinical Videourodynamics. AUA Update Series 2003;XXII(35):278.

9. Aponte MM, Shah SR, Hickling D, et al. Urodynamics for clinically suspected obstruction after anti-incontinence surgery in women. J Urol 2013; 190(2):598–602.

10. Brucker BM, Fong E, Shah S, et al. Urodynamic differences between dysfunctional voiding and primary bladder neck obstruction in women. Urology 2012;80(1):55–60.

11. Lin PJ. Technical advances of interventional fluoroscopy and flat panel image receptor. Health Phys 2008;95(5):650–7.

12. American College of Radiology: ACR Manual on Contrast Media, Version 9. 2013, 9(9): 123. Available at: http://www.acr.org/quality-safety/resources/contrast-manual.

13. Marks B, Vasavada S, Goldman HB. 2282 Contrast concentration does not alter fluoro-urodynamic interpretation. J Urol 2013;189(4):e936.

14. Lee CL, Wunderle K, Vasavada SP, et al. Reduction of radiation during fluoroscopic urodynamics: analysis of quality assurance protocol limiting fluoroscopic images during fluoroscopic urodynamic studies. Urology 2011;78(3):540–3.

15. Herschorn S, Peers G. Videourodynamics. In: Drutz HP, Herschorn S, Diamant NE, editors. Female pelvic medicine and reconstructive pelvic surgery. London: Springer; 2003. p. 107–19.

16. Nitti VW, Tu LM, Gitlin J. Diagnosing bladder outlet obstruction in women. J Urol 1999;161(5):1535–40.

Urodynamics in Stress Incontinence

When Are They Necessary and How Do We Use Them?

Lysanne Campeau, MD, PhD, FRCSC

KEYWORDS

- Stress urinary incontinence • Mixed urinary incontinence • Urodynamics • Cystometry
- Midurethral slings • TVT • TVT-O

KEY POINTS

- Surgical treatment of stress urinary incontinence with retropubic or transobturator midurethral slings offers excellent results with a low risk of adverse events.
- Urodynamics are prudent when the diagnosis of stress urinary incontinence is not confirmed by other investigations or when prior surgical intervention has failed.
- Two recent noninferiority randomized controlled trials did not demonstrate a significant difference in objective and subjective treatment outcome following stress urinary incontinence surgery between women who had a preoperative office evaluation or urodynamic studies.

Urinary incontinence is defined as the "complaint of involuntary loss of urine".[1] Several types of urinary incontinence have been described that may require different treatment approaches. The prevalence of urinary incontinence in women older than 20 years is 25% and increases with age. Half of incontinent women experience stress incontinence alone, and 36% have mixed incontinence.[2] Stress urinary incontinence (SUI) is defined as the "complaint of involuntary loss of urine on effort or physical exertion, or on sneezing and coughing".[1] The diagnosis of SUI in women is based on symptoms and signs as demonstrated on the physical examination or on urodynamic observation in the absence of a detrusor contraction.[3] Stress incontinence may also be diagnosed in the presence of other conditions, such as urinary frequency, urgency, nocturia, or voiding difficulty.[3] Other types of urinary incontinence can coexist with SUI, such as urgency urinary incontinence (UUI), mixed urinary incontinence (MUI), or nocturnal enuresis.

COST OF URODYNAMIC STUDIES

The goal of urodynamic studies (UDS) in women with SUI is to objectively demonstrate the type of urinary incontinence and exclude other diagnoses. Therefore, this assessment may be helpful when the benefits outweigh the costs. The main benefits would be to improve patient outcomes (ie, cure the urinary incontinence) and prevent any adverse events. The costs are related to the invasive nature of the test. It can cause patient embarrassment,[4] pain during and after the test,[5] and urinary tract infections.[6] UDS are expensive, time-consuming evaluations, with costs that vary according to health care systems. A cost-effectiveness study demonstrated that a basic office evaluation was less costly to cure incontinence in a population

Funding Source and Conflict of Interest: Nil.
Division of Urology, Department of Surgery, Jewish General Hospital, Lady Davis Institute for Medical Research, McGill University, 3755 Chemin de la Côte-Sainte-Catherine, Montreal, Quebec H3T 1E2, Canada
E-mail address: lcampeau@jgh.mcgill.ca

Urol Clin N Am 41 (2014) 393–398
http://dx.doi.org/10.1016/j.ucl.2014.05.001

with highly prevalent SUI-only patients.[7] A decision analysis model demonstrated that immediate sling placement for women with pure SUI or MUI was less costly and more effective than basing the treatment decision on the UDS finding.[8] UDS interpretation is subjected to variable reliability and quality, as it is highly operator dependent. Urodynamic testing has the risk of false positives from a series of physiologic and equipment artifacts, which include straining, rectal contraction, or poor pressure transmission.[9] On the other hand, it can result in false negatives if it does not reproduce the patients' symptoms. For instance, 10% to 18% of asymptomatic volunteers have uninhibited detrusor contractions on the urodynamic evaluation; up to 40% of patients with urge incontinence do not show detrusor overactivity on cystometrogram.[10]

URODYNAMIC EVALUATION

UDS can describe a series of different physiologic tests but most commonly refers to the more complete assessment of multichannel cystometry. Simultaneous recording of intravesical and intra-abdominal pressure allows an assessment of bladder sensation, capacity, and compliance, along with the voiding pattern.

Urethral function in a setting of clinical SUI can be better understood during cystometry. It can show a normal urethral closure mechanism or an incompetent one with either urethral relaxation incontinence (leakage in the absence of raised abdominal pressure) or urodynamic stress incontinence (with an increased intra-abdominal pressure). The urethral pressure profile can also be measured along with leak point pressures. The abdominal leak point pressure (ALPP) or the Valsalva leak point pressure (VLPP) is particularly of interest in the urodynamic assessment of SUI, as it establishes the lowest intravesical pressure required to provoke urinary leakage per urethra in the absence of a detrusor contraction (**Fig. 1**).[1]

Certain observations or diagnoses that can coexist with SUI can only be made with the urodynamic evaluation: an overactive detrusor function (with or without incontinence), an abnormal detrusor activity during voiding (detrusor underactivity), or abnormal compliance. Abnormal urethral functions, such as a bladder outlet obstruction or dysfunctional voiding, can only be confirmed during pressure-flow studies.

CLINICAL SCENARIOS

Urodynamics are prudent in scenarios whereby the complete diagnosis of patients cannot be

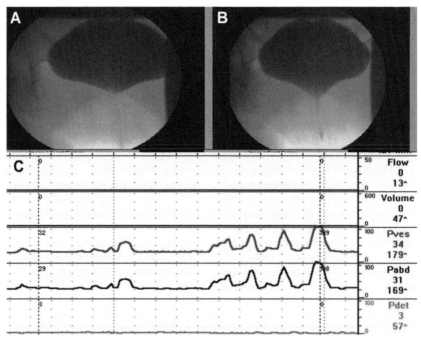

Fig. 1. Urodynamic stress incontinence with hypermobility. (*A*) Cystography at rest. (*B*) Cystography with Valsalva showing contrast leaking in urethra and hypermobility of the bladder neck and urethra. (*C*) Cystometry with sequential increase in generated abdominal pressure, with concomitant increase in vesical pressure. Lowest vesical pressure required to cause leakage per urethra shows ALPP of 109 cm H$_2$O. Pabd, abdominal pressure; Pdet, detrusor pressure; Pves, vesical pressure. (*Courtesy of* Dr Victor Nitti, New York, NY.)

made otherwise, and the diagnosis is required for adequate and safe treatment. The possible scenarios of a woman presenting with a complaint of SUI on history are as follows: (1) The diagnosis of SUI is confirmed by other modalities, and other diagnoses are unlikely based on the assessment. (2) The diagnosis of SUI is confirmed, and other diagnoses are not excluded. (3) The diagnosis of SUI is suspected but not confirmed, and other diagnoses are unlikely based on the assessment. (4) The diagnosis of SUI is suspected but not confirmed, and other diagnoses are not excluded.

The first scenario would be a case whereby clinical stress leakage was demonstrated on the physical examination, and other diagnoses, such as UUI, were not elicited on history or questionnaires, with a normal uroflowmetry and postvoid residual. The second scenario may occur if a patient has symptoms of MUI (complaint of involuntary leakage associated with urgency and also with effort, exertion, sneezing, and coughing) with clinical stress leakage. If the diagnosis of SUI is suspected but not confirmed, it is wise to demonstrate it before considering surgical treatment; this could be achieved with a urodynamic evaluation. Most surgeons would agree that UDS would be useful in the third and fourth scenario without being a question of debate. It is also judicious to consider UDS for recurrent SUI if a prior surgical intervention has failed for better treatment planning.

WHY ARE WE ASKING THE QUESTION?

The necessity of UDS in the clinical management of SUI is being questioned because of the uncertain diagnostic accuracy and associated costs and risks. The diagnostic accuracy of a test can be determined by comparing its test results against a diagnostic gold standard, which defines true disease status. As this does not exist for the clinical entity of SUI, the diagnostic accuracy is extrapolated for the outcomes of SUI treatment after the urodynamic assessment.[11] If urodynamics help guide management and make the right treatment decision to improve patient outcomes, it may, therefore, outweigh the associated costs and risks.

UDS should be performed after formulating specific questions: What information must be obtained? What urodynamic technique is the most appropriate to obtain it?[12] Depending on the urodynamic findings, the management may be altered. The results may indicate if surgical treatment could benefit patients and, if so, guide the preferable surgical option. If the urodynamic results do not suggest that surgical treatment would be indicated, alternative treatment modalities may be considered.

COMPARING OFFICE EVALUATION VERSUS PREOPERATIVE UDS

Two recent noninferiority randomized controlled trials have addressed the question. The Value of Urodynamics prior to Stress Incontinence Surgery randomized 59 women with SUI or stress-predominant MUI to a treatment strategy with or without UDS from different centers. Their study was underpowered because of slow recruitment. The clinical reduction of complaints after 12 months was in favor of the group without urodynamics. Urodynamics did not result in a lower occurrence of de novo urgency.[13] The large multicenter Value of Urodynamic Evaluation (VaLUE) study randomized 630 women planning to undergo surgery for SUI to an office evaluation or urodynamic testing. A provocative stress test was positive for all patients before randomization. After adjusting for the baseline differences between the 2 groups (duration of incontinence; Incontinence Severity Index score; and status with respect to smoking, history of nonsurgical treatment of urinary incontinence, current use of hormone-replacement therapy, and urethral mobility), the treatment success met the noninferiority for office evaluation only at the 1-year follow-up. There were no differences in adverse events outcomes. The preoperative diagnosis was more likely to change after the urodynamic evaluation but did not change the distribution of surgical treatment compared with the office evaluation only.[14] The physician's confidence in the diagnosis improved after UDS but did not correlate with the treatment success.[15] A secondary analysis of the VaLUE trial examined the diagnosis change following UDS and its impact on the treatment plan in efficacy outcomes. The UDS decreased the diagnoses of overactive bladder (OAB)-dry, OAB-wet, and intrinsic sphincter deficiency (ISD) but increased the diagnosis of voiding dysfunction. The number of SUI diagnoses did not change. There was a global treatment plan change in 14% of patients. Surgery was canceled in 1.4%, and the procedure changed in 5.4%. These changes were not associated with more successful outcomes but increased the odds of the treatment of urgency at 3 and 12 months postoperatively.[16] The findings of these 2 trials, which included patients with very strict selection criteria managed by expert hands, may not be generalizable to the wide clinical population.

Clement and colleagues[11] reported a Cochrane review on the value of urodynamic investigations in the treatment of urinary incontinence. They included eight 2-arm randomized controlled trials.

Three of these were done in women with predominant SUI, including those 2 previously mentioned trials. They demonstrated no statistically significant difference in the primary outcome of urinary incontinence between women undergoing an office evaluation or urodynamic investigations. Another meta-analysis that gathered the results of these 2 trials and another unpublished study to compare the outcomes after surgery for SUI found no statistical difference in subjective or objective cure/improvement. Voiding dysfunction was similar in both groups, and there was a trend for continued treatment of urgency in the office-evaluation group.[17] Meta-analyses offer a useful global perspective of the highest quality of evidence by grouping patients from several high-quality trials and comparing outcomes between many patients. Although offering the advantage of a higher power from a larger sample, it brings in the limitation of a potentially more heterogeneous group and obscuring a more individualized approach.

TYPES OF URINARY INCONTINENCE

Symptoms can help elucidate the type of incontinence present. Certain patients have stress-predominant incontinence symptoms. There is also a group of patients with insensible incontinence, as "the complaint of urinary incontinence where the woman has been unaware of how it occurred".[1] These patients will benefit from urodynamic evaluation, as urodynamic SUI is the most prevalent finding in this population and could be treated accordingly.[18] Other patients may be unable to determine the predominant type between UUI and SUI and, therefore, fall in the category of MUI. Heinonen and colleagues[19] report a poorer short-term and long-term outcome in women with MUI who underwent a tension-free vaginal tape (TVT) procedure without preoperative urodynamic testing, as compared with women with SUI alone (69% vs 97% at 36 months). However, their long-term success of women with SUI 10 years after the TVT procedure without preoperative urodynamics was quite high (90% objective and 78% subjective cure rates). Patients with MUI fair worse after a midurethral sling procedure as compared with SUI alone. A systematic review and meta-analysis of randomized trials and prospective studies showed a subjective cure rate of 56.4% at 34.9 ± 22.9 months' follow-up. Women with MUI did not have any significant difference in subjective and UUI cure rates between the transobturator and retropubic approach.[20]

SELECTION OF SURGICAL TECHNIQUE

The Trial of Mid-Urethral Slings (TOMUS) randomized 597 women with a positive urinary stress test to undergo a midurethral sling through either a retropubic or transobturator route. They all had a preoperative urodynamic evaluation blinded to the surgeon, and the urodynamic stress leakage was not required. There were no objective or subjective differences in treatment success between both groups, even when adjusted for VLPP or maximum urethral closure pressure at 12 or 24 months.[21,22]

Lemack and colleagues[23] analyzed the preoperative standardized UDS performed on the participants of the Stress Incontinence Treatment Efficacy Trial that randomized patients to Burch colposuspension or pubovaginal sling. No UDS findings were associated with an increased risk of voiding dysfunction (defined as the use of a catheter or the need for reoperation) in either group.

The demonstration of urodynamically proven MUI may not be a prognostic factor for treatment success according to the type of procedure. In fact, a prospective cohort of women with urodynamically proven MUI treated with a midurethral sling did not have any significant differences in postoperative symptoms between those who underwent TVT or tension-free vaginal tape obturator (TVT-O). However, those who underwent TVT had a lower risk of having detrusor overactivity on UDS after 12 months.[24]

The presence of ISD or urethral mobility (as demonstrated with the cotton swab test) provides important information about the nature of the stress incontinence. The value of the maximal urethral closure pressure (MUCP) or the ALPP does not correlate with each other,[25] and both urodynamic parameters may not correlate with urethral mobility.[26,27] In the TOMUS trial, body mass index and detrusor pressure at maximal flow (PdetQmax) positively correlated with the VLPP and MUCP. Pad weight and age negatively correlated with MUCP, whereas the duration of incontinence negatively correlated with the VLPP.[28] A randomized study of TVT versus Monarc found that the retropubic approach was more effective in women with urodynamic SUI and ISD as defined by a MUCP of 20 cm H_2O or less or a VLPP of 60 cm H_2O or less, with no mention of urethral mobility.[29] The value of the VLPP in a retrospective study of 204 women who underwent TVT-O did not impact the treatment outcome or self-reported quality of life postoperatively.[30]

SUMMARY

The decision to use urodynamics as a diagnostic tool should be made according the expertise and the ability of the surgeon to efficiently use this information for planning SUI treatment. As a surgeon gains experience and training to interpret urodynamic tracings, it becomes more valuable. For the same reason, the experienced surgeon may become more selective for patients who would benefit from urodynamic evaluation and use it more judiciously. The specialty-trained surgeon will likely treat patients of higher complexity who may benefit from the additional evidence gained from a urodynamic evaluation. They, therefore, manage fewer patients with uncomplicated SUI. Their expertise and clinical experience could potentially allow them to treat and manage patients with simple SUI with or without preoperative UDS. This might explain why the 2 major randomized clinical trials did not identify any significant difference in outcome with or without preoperative urodynamics for the treatment of SUI. Ultimately, the necessity and value of a urodynamic evaluation will vary according to each surgeon's expertise and each patient's unique type of incontinence, severity, and concomitant urinary symptoms.

REFERENCES

1. Haylen BT, de Ridder D, Freeman RM, et al. An International Urogynecological Association (IUGA)/International Continence Society (ICS) joint report on the terminology for female pelvic floor dysfunction. Neurourol Urodyn 2010;29(1):4–20.
2. Hannestad YS, Rortveit G, Sandvik H, et al. A community-based epidemiological survey of female urinary incontinence: the Norwegian EPINCONT Study. J Clin Epidemiol 2000;53(11):1150–7.
3. Abrams P, Cardozo L, Fall M, et al. The standardisation of terminology of lower urinary tract function: report from the standardisation sub-committee of the International Continence Society. Neurourol Urodyn 2002;21(2):167–78.
4. Neustaedter EG, Milne J, Shorten K, et al. How well informed are women who undergo urodynamic testing? Neurourol Urodyn 2011;30(4):572–7.
5. Yokoyama T, Nozaki K, Nose H, et al. Tolerability and morbidity of urodynamic testing: a questionnaire-based study. Urology 2005;66(1):74–6.
6. Foon R, Toozs-Hobson P, Latthe P. Prophylactic antibiotics to reduce the risk of urinary tract infections after urodynamic studies. Cochrane Database Syst Rev 2012;(10). CD008224. Available at: http://onlinelibrary.wiley.com/doi/10.1002/14651858.CD008224.pub2/abstract.
7. Weber AM, Taylor RJ, Wei JT, et al. The cost-effectiveness of preoperative testing (basic office assessment vs urodynamics) for stress urinary incontinence in women. BJU Int 2002;89(4):356–63.
8. Geisler JP, Drenchko R. Cost-effectiveness of urodynamics testing in women with predominant stress incontinence symptoms. Obstet Gynecol 2014;123(Suppl 1):197S.
9. Hogan S, Gammie A, Abrams P. Urodynamic features and artefacts. Neurourol Urodyn 2012;31(7):1104–17.
10. Mahfouz W, Afraa T, Campeau L, et al. Normal urodynamic parameters in women. Int Urogynecol J 2012;23(3):269–77.
11. Clement Keiran D, Lapitan Marie Carmela M, Omar Muhammad I, et al. Urodynamic studies for management of urinary incontinence in children and adults. Cochrane Database Syst Rev 2013;(10):CD003195.
12. Winters JC, Dmochowski RR, Goldman HB, et al. Urodynamic studies in adults: AUA/SUFU guideline. J Urol 2012;188(Suppl 6):2464–72.
13. van Leijsen SA, Kluivers KB, Mol BW, et al. Can preoperative urodynamic investigation be omitted in women with stress urinary incontinence? A non-inferiority randomized controlled trial. Neurourol Urodyn 2012;31(7):1118–23.
14. Nager CW, Brubaker L, Litman HJ, et al. A randomized trial of urodynamic testing before stress-incontinence surgery. N Engl J Med 2012;366(21):1987–97.
15. Zimmern P, Litman H, Nager C, et al. Pre-operative urodynamics in women with stress urinary incontinence increases physician confidence, but does not improve outcomes. Neurourol Urodyn 2014;33(3):302–6.
16. Sirls LT, Richter HE, Litman HJ, et al. The effect of urodynamic testing on clinical diagnosis, treatment plan and outcomes in women undergoing stress urinary incontinence surgery. J Urol 2013;189(1):204–9.
17. Rachaneni S, Latthe P. Urodynamic before stress incontinence surgery – a systematic review and meta-analysis. Barcelona (Spain): International Continence Society; 2013.
18. Brucker BM, Fong E, Kaefer D, et al. Urodynamic findings in women with insensible incontinence. Int J Urol 2013;20(4):429–33.
19. Heinonen P, Ala-Nissilä S, Kiilholma P, et al. Tension-free vaginal tape procedure without preoperative urodynamic examination: long-term outcome. Int J Urol 2012;19(11):1003–9.
20. Jain P, Jirschele K, Botros S, et al. Effectiveness of midurethral slings in mixed urinary incontinence: a systematic review and meta-analysis. Int Urogynecol J 2011;22(8):923–32.

21. Richter HE, Albo ME, Zyczynski HM, et al. Retropubic versus transobturator midurethral slings for stress incontinence. N Engl J Med 2010;362(22):2066–76.

22. Albo ME, Litman HJ, Richter HE, et al. Treatment success of retropubic and transobturator mid urethral slings at 24 months. J Urol 2012;188(6):2281–7.

23. Lemack GE, Krauss S, Litman H, et al. Normal preoperative urodynamic testing does not predict voiding dysfunction after Burch colposuspension versus pubovaginal sling. J Urol 2008;180(5):2076–80.

24. Athanasiou S, Grigoriadis T, Giannoulis G, et al. Midurethral slings for women with urodynamic mixed incontinence: what to expect? Int Urogynecol J 2013;24(3):393–9.

25. McGuire EJ, Fitzpatrick CC, Wan J, et al. Clinical assessment of urethral sphincter function. J Urol 1993;150(5 Pt 1):1452–4.

26. Fleischmann N, Flisser AJ, Blaivas JG, et al. Sphincteric urinary incontinence: relationship of vesical leak point pressure, urethral mobility and severity of incontinence. J Urol 2003;169(3):999–1002.

27. Bump RC, Coates KW, Cundiff GW, et al. Diagnosing intrinsic sphincteric deficiency: comparing urethral closure pressure, urethral axis, and Valsalva leak point pressures. Am J Obstet Gynecol 1997;177(2):303–10.

28. Chai TC, Huang L, Kenton K, et al. Association of baseline urodynamic measures of urethral function with clinical, demographic, and other urodynamic variables in women prior to undergoing midurethral sling surgery. Neurourol Urodyn 2012;31(4):496–501.

29. Schierlitz L, Dwyer PL, Rosamilia A, et al. Effectiveness of tension-free vaginal tape compared with transobturator tape in women with stress urinary incontinence and intrinsic sphincter deficiency: a randomized controlled trial. Obstet Gynecol 2008;112(6):1253–61.

30. Ryu JG, Yu SH, Jeong SH, et al. Transobturator tape for female stress urinary incontinence: preoperative Valsalva leak point pressure is not related to cure rate or quality of life improvement. Korean J Urol 2014;55(4):265–9.

Urodynamics in Male LUTS

When Are They Necessary and How Do We Use Them?

Lindsey Cox, MD[a],*, William I. Jaffe, MD[b]

KEYWORDS

- Urodynamics • Benign prostatic enlargement • Benign prostatic obstruction
- Lower urinary tract symptoms • Transurethral resection of the prostate

KEY POINTS

- There is no effective method of diagnosing benign prostatic obstruction (BPO) other than pressure flow urodynamics (PFUDS).
- The outcomes for surgical outlet reduction are worse for patients who do not demonstrate outlet obstruction on PFUDS.
- Patients with male lower urinary tract symptoms (MLUTS) prefer a shared problem-solving and decision-making model when evaluating treatment strategies.

INTRODUCTION

Lower urinary tract symptoms (LUTS) are a frequently encountered constellation of symptoms that consist of deviations from the usual storage and emptying functions of the lower urinary tract. The term *male lower urinary tract symptoms* describes an older male presenting with LUTS and implies no particular cause of these symptoms. This index patient has been depicted as a middle-aged or elderly man (often >50 years) with bothersome dysfunction of urinary storage, voiding, and/or the postmicturition period that often consists of a combination of frequency, urgency, nocturia, as well as hesitancy, weak stream, and feeling of incomplete emptying. Because an enlarged prostate gland that causes obstruction of the urinary outflow is the most likely cause of these symptoms, the term *benign prostatic hyperplasia*

(BPH) has historically been attached to these symptoms. More recently, the terms *benign prostatic enlargement* (BPE) and *benign prostatic obstruction* (BPO) have largely taken the place of BPH, a term limited to the histologic proliferation of smooth muscle and epithelial cells in the prostate gland. It is difficult to define what characterizes clinically significant MLUTS, but patient-reported bother certainly plays the central role in clinical decision making. Because bother, prostate size, and urodynamically proven outflow obstruction are not always well correlated, it is not possible to make assumptions that LUTS occurring in men are explained by BPO caused by BPE. Therefore, the identification of causes of non-BPO MLUTS is a key component of each step of the evaluation of these patients. For the purposes of this article, all patients who present like the index patient are considered: with bothersome MLUTS without known cause, but

Disclosures and Conflicts of Interest: None.
[a] Female Pelvic Medicine and Reconstructive Surgery, Department of Urology, University of Michigan, 3875 Taubman Center, 1500 East Medical Center Drive, SPC 5330, Ann Arbor, MI 48109-5330, USA; [b] Division of Urology, Department of Surgery, Perelman Center for Advanced Medicine, University of Pennsylvania, West Pavilion, 3rd Floor, 3400 Civic Center Boulevard, Philadelphia, PA 19104, USA
* Corresponding author.
E-mail address: lmenchen@med.umich.edu

Urol Clin N Am 41 (2014) 399–407
http://dx.doi.org/10.1016/j.ucl.2014.04.009
0094-0143/14/$ – see front matter © 2014 Elsevier Inc. All rights reserved.

statistically likely to be caused by BPO. Although the focus is on the role of urodynamics (UDS) in adding value to the evaluation of the patient with MLUTS suggestive of BPO, the value of UDS in identifying other causes of LUTS is also considered.

Describing the epidemiology and natural history of the problem of MLUTS is somewhat complicated by the way in which MLUTS is defined because of the use of data from studies of patients with BPH. There are biases present when extrapolating data from clinical trial populations, and testing for BPE, BPO, or histologic BPH would be invasive and costly; therefore, prostate and/or outlet obstruction is not necessarily the cause of LUTS in all patients in these calculations. It is reasonable to examine the efficiency and effectiveness of care for patients with MLUTS by starting with the evaluation of an undifferentiated symptomatic index patient, not the patient with definitive MLUTS with BPO. It is accepted that MLUTS is a common problem that deserves our attention. In the United States, moderate to severe LUTS was approximated to occur in 6.7 million of the 27 million men aged 50 to 79 years in the year 2000.[1] In the United Kingdom between 1992 and 2001, the prevalence of LUTS in a general practice population was around 3.5% for men in their 40s, increasing to greater than 30% for men older than 85 years.[2] In Sweden, a population study of 40,000 men aged 45 to 79 years showed 18.5% of men having moderate symptoms and 4.8% having severe LUTS.[3] Wei and colleagues[1] also note that the significant variation in the management of patients with MLUTS is a concern for the quality of care for this condition.

The focus on when UDS is necessary in MLUTS and how it is used boils down to the value that these studies add for shared decision making with patients and for determining the effectiveness of therapy. Educating patients on the various tradeoffs within treatment choices helps meet the objectives for treating MLUTS: improving patients' quality of life by relief of bothersome symptoms, avoiding morbidity, and potentially slowing disease progression. Ideally, each individual could be accurately diagnosed, the outcomes of conservative management or active treatments could be predicted, and the chance of success could be maximized while minimizing adverse events, costly repeat evaluations, re-treatment, and failures—thus theoretically improving both patient and provider satisfaction. Avoiding the morbidities of BPO including acute or chronic urinary retention, the need for catheterization, and the attendant problems therein, urinary tract infections (UTIs), obstructive uropathy, and urinary calculi

should also be considered benefits of appropriate treatment. The authors' objective is to define the role of UDS in the current diagnostic algorithm and treatment of MLUTS in general, and especially MLUTS that is nonneurogenic, not associated with malignancy or other comorbid conditions, and not caused by infection, trauma, medications, radiation, or surgery.

Clinical guidelines are a valuable source of aggregated data and current expert opinion on the evaluation and treatment of MLUTS. The American Urological Association (AUA) and has published updated guidelines in the past 3 years that discuss the role of UDS in the diagnosis and workup of MLUTS, especially in the context of BPO.[4] The AUA/SUFU (Society of Urodynamics, Female Pelvic Mecidine and Urogenital Reconstruction) Guidelines on Urodynamics in Adults also addresses this issue.[5] In addition, the 6th International Consultation on Urologic Diseases (ICUD) consensus document was developed in 2005 and later summarized by Abrams and colleagues[6] providing the basis for many of the subsequent algorithms. It is useful to examine these guidelines and review the evidence that led to their adoption so that one can apply these guidelines to the appropriate populations in practice. These guidelines characterize the specific index patient to which they apply, and understanding when UDS is recommended and also where patients come to intervention points with multiple options in an algorithm, or fall off the algorithm altogether, can help define when urodynamic evaluations provide value.

The 6th International Consultation on New Developments in Prostate Cancer & Prostate Diseases took place in 2005, and the consensus document on "Male Lower Urinary Tract Dysfunction: Evaluation and Management" was published in 2006 and summarized by Abrams and colleagues[6] in 2009. The guidelines on "Evaluation and Treatment of Lower Urinary Tract Symptoms in Older Men" delineate a basic evaluation of the index patient including history, assessment of symptoms and bother, physical examination and digital rectal examination, urinalysis, serum prostate-specific antigen levels, and frequency-volume charts. For patients considering active treatment, the panel also recommends symptom quantification with validated questionnaires (I-PSS, ICIQ-MLUTS, and DAN-PSS-1), flow rate recording, postvoid residual (PVR), prostate imaging via ultrasonography, upper tract imaging and endoscopy under certain circumstances, and pressure flow studies (PFSs), which are recommended before invasive therapy in men with a maximum urinary flow rate (Q_{max}) greater than 10 mL/s. The argument made is that flow rates above this level raise suspicion of causes of LUTS other than obstruction and patients who do not have obstruction are less likely to benefit from outlet reduction procedures.

The AUA guidelines on the Management of Benign Prostatic Hyperplasia (BPH) have undergone multiple revisions since they were initially presented in 1994, most recently in 2010,[4] and are available at www.auanet.org/content/guidelines-and-quality-care/clinical-guidelines.cfm?sub=bph. The algorithms presented in the guidelines were adopted from the ICUD document and again include the use of PFSs when the patient is being offered minimally invasive or invasive surgical treatment and the evaluation does not clearly indicate obstruction, that is, the maximum flow rate on uroflowmetry is greater than 10 mL/s. The committee notes that PFSs are an optional part of the evaluation, which categorizes their use as having the highest level of flexibility with regard to application of guideline statements.

The AUA also addresses MLUTS in the AUA/SUFU Guidelines on Urodynamics in Adults.[5] The panel recommends uroflowmetry for the initial diagnosis and ongoing management of MLUTS with a grade C level of evidence and makes note of the pitfall of variability of the measurements, as well as the risks of false positives and false negatives. The panel separately addresses cystometry and PFSs. Multichannel filling cystometry is noted to have little evidence for use in the management of patients with LUTS, with expert opinion cited as the basis for recommending that cystometry may be performed to identify detrusor overactivity (DO) or poor compliance when invasive/irreversible treatments are being considered. The panel recommends PFSs as a standard with grade B evidence, stating that they should be performed when diagnosing obstruction is important, especially when considering invasive treatment. The panel notes that the current scientific evidence, although not without variability, does point to PFS-confirmed obstruction as a predictor of improved outcomes from treatment. The guideline also specifies that the urodynamic study itself should be discussed with the patient with regard to its benefits, shortcomings, and possible complications.

The European Association of Urology (EAU) had previously published guidelines under the title "Assessment, Therapy and Follow-Up of Men with Lower Urinary Tract Symptoms Suggestive of Benign Prostatic Obstruction (BPH Guidelines)." These were most recently updated in 2013 and summarized by Oelke and colleagues[7] in their article "EAU Guidelines on the Treatment and Follow-up of Non-neurogenic Male Lower Urinary Tract Symptoms Including Benign Prostatic Obstruction." The updated document takes a symptom- and treatment-based approach and does not delineate specific guidelines regarding the workup of patients with MLUTS.

McNicholas and colleagues[8] convey a similar outlook in *Campbell-Walsh Urology, Tenth Edition*: "If the initial evaluation, flow rate, and PVR urine volume are not sufficiently suggestive of BOO, further urodynamic assessment by PFSs should be considered, especially if an invasive treatment is considered (ie, surgery) or if surgical treatment has failed."

Describing the pathophysiology of MLUTS and the details of each of the treatment options available is beyond the scope of this article; however, in the context of choosing when to use UDS evaluations, the article discusses how to define and diagnose the cause of the symptoms of MLUTS and how treatment outcomes have been evaluated using urodynamic data.

URODYNAMIC PRINCIPLES

The most basic tenet of UDS evaluation is that of prospectively formulating the urodynamic questions. Lenherr and Clemens[9] describe in detail the compilation of a thorough evaluation of all known clinical, laboratory, and radiologic data to choose appropriate studies that are targeted to answering a specific question and advocate having a clinician present to ensure that the study is well annotated and reproduces the patient's symptoms.

Most algorithms begin with the option of performing noninvasive evaluations including uroflowmetry and PVR. Uroflowmetry ultimately can detect only the rate of urine flow with no way to distinguish underactive detrusor, outlet obstruction, or a combination of both[10] and some patients can generate what is considered a normal flow in the face of obstruction, which is the cause of their symptoms.

Invasive tests include cystometry, PFS, sphincter electromyography (EMG), urethral function tests/profilometry, and videourodynamics (VUDS). Invasive UDS testing usually involves the use of a double- or triple-lumen urethral catheter to fill the bladder and record vesical and (in the case of triple lumen catheters) urethral pressures. The addition of an abdominal pressure sensor (typically placed rectally) to multichannel UDS provides a measurement of abdominal pressure and allows for the subtraction of this value from the vesical pressure in order to calculate the actual detrusor pressure. Cystometry is the recording of vesical or detrusor pressures during filling to evaluate the storage phase of lower urinary tract function. Several useful diagnostic features of cystometry apply to the MLUTS population. Involuntary detrusor contractions or DO can be identified, and during the study, the clinician can correlate this phenomenon with patient-reported symptoms of urgency and urgency incontinence. DO is found in more than 50% of men with prostatic obstruction, and in one investigation of 1418 men with LUTS, the prevalence of DO on UDS increased continuously from 51.4% in Schäfer class 0 to 83.3% in Schäfer class V.[11]

Bladder compliance is an important storage parameter to consider in all patients, and although less commonly seen in the MLUTS population, loss of bladder compliance is a finding that would affect management decisions. Cystometric capacity can be measured and correlated with functional capacity on frequency-volume charts. Along with sensation, capacity measurements can inform preoperative counseling in patients with decreased sensation and large capacity as well as in patients with a large sensory component driving frequency and urgency symptoms. Incontinence is a less frequent symptom associated with MLUTS, and the finding of involuntary loss of urine during UDS for MLUTS in a patient considering interventions that may have incontinence as a potential adverse event is a useful device for counseling.

PFSs have the unique feature of being able to determine the detrusor pressure simultaneously with voiding, which can differentiate an underactive detrusor from a well-functioning detrusor generating high pressures with low flow. The abdominal pressure sensor can determine the contribution of Valsalva or abdominal straining to voiding, and this can be correlated with hesitancy and difficulty initiating voiding. For patients who are unable to voluntarily void during UDS because of situational factors or discomfort, the diagnosis of obstruction becomes confounded. If the patient cannot mount a detrusor contraction with the catheter in place, removing the UDS catheter to allow for void also removes the ability to determine vesical and detrusor pressures during voiding. Noting the detrusor pressures during attempts at voiding to judge contractility and using fluoroscopy to delineate the level of obstruction (eg, a stricture or bladder neck contracture that is similar in caliber to the urodynamic catheter) can be helpful.

By the International Continence Society (ICS) definitions, detrusor contractility falls into 3 categories, acontractile, underactive, and normal.[12] Contractility can be quantified by several formulas such as the bladder contractility index (pdetQ$_{max}$ + 5Q$_{max}$, with strong ≥150, normal 100–150, or weak ≤100) or absolute detrusor pressure cutoffs for normal values, which have been used in prior research on the contribution of detrusor underactivity to MLUTS, but recent attention has been placed on the ambiguity of this term and its definition/diagnosis.[13] The importance of this urodynamic finding is illustrated in the similar presentations, but different PFSs for the 2 patients in **Figs. 1** and **2**.

Obstruction of urinary outflow has been extensively studied and nomograms and formulas, including the commonly used bladder outlet obstruction index (pdetQ$_{max}$ − 2Q$_{max}$, with obstructed ≥40, equivocal 20–40, and unobstructed ≤20) have been developed to diagnose and quantify the severity of outlet obstruction on PFSs. The ICS nomogram[14] was developed as a provisional standardized definition for obstruction, and the developers reference its similarities to the Abrams-Griffiths and Spangberg nomograms and the Schäfer diagram using linear Passive Urethral Resistance Relation (linPURR) and its overlapping characteristics with the urethral resistance factor (URA) and two dimensional CHESS classification methods at low to moderate flow rates. The authors advocate using this nomogram as the standard in the MLUTS population. Noninvasive techniques for making the diagnosis of obstruction were summarized in an earlier version of this article, with varying degrees of sensitivity and specificity, and none of these have come into common clinical use.[15]

UDS can suggest detrusor sphincter dyssynergia or bradykinesia on EMG or fluoroscopy (in the case of VUDS) in a population that has no known neurologic diagnoses and may prompt neurologic evaluation. These conditions are not as common in this population, but some neurologic conditions may present with bothersome urinary tract symptoms. These patients benefit from accurate diagnosis and avoidance of treatment of prostatic obstruction. It is also uncommon to find pseudodyssynergia on EMG or fluoroscopy diagnosing dysfunctional voiding as the sole cause of MLUTS; however, refractory LUTS in a younger male may be related to pelvic floor dysfunction, and treatment would again diverge from the typical MLUTS pathway for older patients.

Along with PFSs that suggest obstruction, radiologic imaging of the lower urinary tract can help define the anatomic location of the obstruction and provide insight into the pathophysiology of the patient's symptoms. Obstruction can occur at the bladder neck as in primary bladder neck obstruction, in the prostatic urethra from prostatic enlargement, in the membranous urethra with

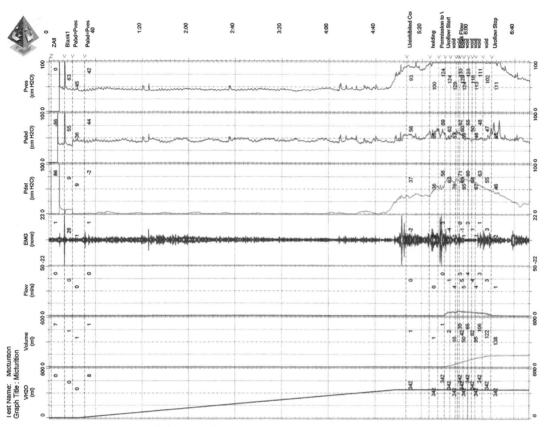

Fig. 1. A 78-year-old man with diabetes mellitus, AUA symptom index 22. Poor emptying, decreased stream, frequency/urgency/nocturia, on terazosin/finasteride, digital rectal exam (DRE) 40 g, Q_{max} on uroflow = 10.2 mL/s, PVR 172 mL, and PFUDS reveals high pressure, low flow, which indicates obstruction.

dysfunctional voiding, or anywhere along the urethra in the case of stricture. Fluoroscopic voiding images can rule out vesicoureteral reflux and other anatomic abnormalities. Fluoroscopy provides the ability to detect bladder diverticula, which can alter pressure and storage characteristics, as well as bladder calculi, both of which can alter the surgical management for these patients.

It cannot be overstated that answering UDS questions with studies that reproduce the patients' bothersome symptoms is the key to defining the pathophysiology that accompanies bother so that this entity can be targeted for therapy. When this therapy is invasive, irreversible and potentially morbid, or costly, PFUDS can be used to accurately target the cause of the patient's symptoms.

Guidelines leave a significant portion of the decision making to the provider to decide when UDS is necessary. In addition to the aforementioned patients, the following scenarios would generally warrant consideration of invasive urodynamic testing: the elderly, especially if there are concerns for limitations in history taking or possible prior surgeries or instrumentation; those

in the younger range of the index patient, or younger[16]; patients with urinary retention and unable to complete uroflowmetry; patients whose symptoms do not correlate with noninvasive findings, or whose symptoms arouse any suspicion of neurologic components to voiding dysfunction and patients with confounding conditions that could affect bladder function (severe diabetes, previous radiation or pelvic surgery, previous spine surgery); patients with MLUTS and incontinence; and patients who have failed prior invasive treatments, because it has been shown that a significant number of these failures are found to have detrusor underactivity.[17]

The risks of UDS include UTI, transient hematuria, patient distress/discomfort or difficulty voiding after instrumentation, and vasovagal syncope as well as variable reproducibility (the equivalent of false positives and false negatives).[18–20] UTI rates are reported as less than 15%, and AUA best practice recommends antimicrobial prophylaxis only with risk factors present.[21] There have been several studies that survey patients regarding the distress/discomfort and embarrassment of UDS

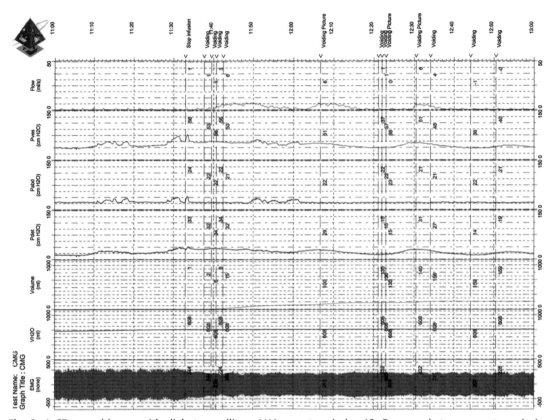

Fig. 2. A 67-year old man with diabetes mellitus, AUA symptom index 18. Decreased stream, on tamsulosin, digital rectal exam (DRE) 30 g, Q_{max} on uroflow = 6 mL/s, PVR 230 mL, PFUDS reveals attempts at voiding with very low detrusor pressures, which indicates detrusor underactivity.

evaluations. Scarpero and colleagues[22] showed that 95% of patients would undergo UDS again if indicated, with levels of pain and embarrassment as expected or less than expected in 90% and 93% of patients, respectively. Ku and colleagues[23] demonstrated that although males (n = 71) had slightly higher pain scores than females (n = 137), these scores were still low overall, with a mean of 3.1 out of 10. UDS is a low-risk evaluation with good tolerability.

ROLE OF UDS

The discussion so far leaves us with the question of how do we use them? There is an increasing body of literature that defines the roles that patients wish to take in their health care decision making. Deber and colleagues[24] surveyed more than 2700 patients including 678 with BPH on their preferred level of autonomy; the vast majority desired a shared model in which patients participated both in problem solving and decision making. There is also evidence of heterogeneity in the treatment characteristics that determine

treatment preference in patients seeking care for MLUTS[25] and that new information regarding treatments can alter patient preferences.[26] Patients who desire education about their condition may have a strong interest in the results of UDS and may prefer to defer decisions on surgical intervention until they can be informed by this type of testing. MLUTS is a chronic condition, and in seeking quality-of-life improvement, we must be sensitive to the patient's goals for treatment, avoid assumptions, and reduce variability, all of which can perhaps be enhanced using UDS.

A commitment to patient-centered health care delivery also demands that interventions be judged on patient-reported outcomes and the patient's perception of success. Research on MLUTS treatments have often used UDS evaluations as part of protocols and have used relief of outlet obstruction as a measure of success, with reporting of increasing flow, decreasing voiding pressure, and decreasing PVR as outcomes. This method has allowed comparisons of treatment modalities and benchmarks for new therapies. These are the parameters on which patients can be counseled and expectations can be set, which would be the basis for their later perceptions of success.

Patients, providers, and payors are interested in predicting successful outcomes of treatment. In a 1994 editorial arguing for the use of PFSs to evaluate MLUTS, Abrams[27] summarized the evidence of several series, including his own, and concluded that failure rates after outlet reduction by transurethral resection of the prostate prostatectomy were higher in those who did not have evidence of obstruction on PFSs, those who had DO, and those who had detrusor underactivity. There are several more contemporary studies that also relate urodynamic diagnoses to successful outcome of outlet reduction procedures. Tanaka and colleagues[28] reported that in 92 patients undergoing transurethral resection of prostate (TURP), a composite outcome for efficacy showed excellent or good results for patients with bladder outlet obstruction (57% of their population on PFSs); still good results for efficacy for patients without outlet obstruction, even with detrusor underactivity; but less efficacy in patients without outlet obstruction with DO. This report suggests that in patients without clear outlet obstruction with possible DO, cystometry and PFUDS can help avoid surgical failures. Similar findings were reported previously by Machino and colleagues[29] when reporting on 62 men undergoing TURP; successful outcome of TURP was not statistically significantly different for those with and without definitive obstruction, but for those with equivocal values for obstruction and DO, success rates fell. Urodynamic obstruction has also been shown to have a useful relationship with symptom improvement from TURP in a case series by van Venrooij

and colleagues.[30] The investigators showed that symptom improvement in unobstructed and equivocal men undergoing TURP was around 70% of that in the obstructed group. This information is helpful in setting expectations for symptom improvement for men with and without obstruction who have chosen surgical treatment and is summarized in **Table 1**.

Discussion of the value of a diagnostic test includes analysis of the cost, both for the individual and society. These costs for an individual UDS evaluation are not inconsequential and should be weighed with possible increases and decreases in the overall cost of caring for patients with MLUTS. Potential cost benefits that may stem from better diagnostic information include decreasing trial-and-error therapy, not only by identifying patients with non-BPO MLUTS and avoiding the cost of unnecessary medications and surgery but also by identifying patients with severe symptoms and proven obstruction that may benefit from early surgical intervention to avoid the cascade effect: many years of medical therapy, then minor surgery, then major surgery. DiSantostefano and colleagues[31] investigated the cost and effectiveness of 6 different treatments for BPH with a 20-year decision analytical model and found that the cost of combination therapy exceeded that of surgical therapy at around 10 years and that the cost difference was especially pronounced in younger men (**Fig. 3**). The investigators note that risk aversion and patient preferences likely play a key role in evaluating which treatment is best for an individual. Finally, UDS with improved counseling could result in more informed patients with care that meets expectations.

Table 1
Urodynamic obstruction as a predictor of success after outlet reduction

Study, Year	Subjects (N)	Outcomes	
Tanaka et al,[28] 2006	92 men undergoing TURP linPURR 0–1 (37) linPURR 2–3 (38) linPURR 4–6 (17)	Excellent/good composite outcome (%) 62.2 84.2 88.2	
Machino et al,[29] 2002	62 men undergoing TURP Equivocal − detrusor instability (21) Equivocal + detrusor instability (7) Obstructed − detrusor instability (13) Obstructed +detrusor instability (21)	Excellent/good composite outcome (%) 82 29 54 88	
van Venrooij et al,[30] 2003	93 men undergoing TURP Unobstructed/equivocal (34) Obstructed (59)	Median flow rate reduction (mL/s) 7.8 11	Median symptom index reduction 10 14

Data from Refs.[28–30]

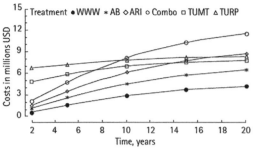

Fig. 3. Expected costs for each treatment over time based on 2004 costs and 3% discount rate: cohort of 1000 men aged 65 years. The plot assumes switching among pharmaceuticals and watchful waiting. AB, α-blockers; ARI, 5 alpha reductase inhibitor; combo, combined pharmacotherapy; TUMT, transurethral microwave therapy; TURP, transurethral resection of prostate; WWW, watchful waiting. (*From* DiSantostefano R, Biddle A, Lavelle J. An evaluation of the economic costs and patient-related consequences of treatments for benign prostatic hyperplasia. Br J Urol 2006;97:1012; with permission.)

SUMMARY

UDS adds value to the evaluation and management of patients with MLUTS when providers are critically assessing treatment strategies and desire the most definitive information. PFUDS offers the best available data to educate patients considering invasive therapy and allows the provider to combine their skills and knowledge with confidence in the diagnosis to realistically engage in shared decision making. The authors see PFUDS as a useful tool to ensure that patients are appropriately selected for irreversible and potentially morbid treatments and to improve satisfaction with outcomes. As new therapies emerge and accepted modalities are modified, large well-designed studies that identify pretreatment urodynamic parameters that are useful for selecting patients for specific modalities are needed to improve the delivery of care for patients with MLUTS.

REFERENCES

1. Wei JT, Calhoun E, Jacobsen SJ. Urologic diseases in America project: benign prostatic hyperplasia. J Urol 2005;173(4):1256–61. http://dx.doi.org/10.1097/01.ju.0000155709.37840.fe.
2. Logie J, Clifford GM, Farmer RD. Incidence, prevalence and management of lower urinary tract symptoms in men in the UK. Br J Urol 2005;95(4):557–62. http://dx.doi.org/10.1111/j.1464-410X.2005.05339.x.
3. Andersson SO, Rashidkhani B, Karlberg L, et al. Prevalence of lower urinary tract symptoms in men aged 45-79 years: a population-based study of 40 000 Swedish men. Br J Urol 2004;94(3):327–31. http://dx.doi.org/10.1111/j.1464-410X.2004.04930.x.
4. McVary KT, Roehrborn CG, Avins AL, et al. Update on AUA guideline on the management of benign prostatic hyperplasia. J Urol 2011;185(5):1793–803. http://dx.doi.org/10.1016/j.juro.2011.01.074.
5. Winters JC, Dmochowski RR, Goldman HB, et al. Urodynamic studies in adults: AUA/SUFU guideline. J Urol 2012;188(Suppl 6):2464–72. http://dx.doi.org/10.1016/j.juro.2012.09.081.
6. Abrams P, Chapple C, Khoury S, et al. Evaluation and treatment of lower urinary tract symptoms in older men. J Urol 2009;181(4):1779–87. http://dx.doi.org/10.1016/j.juro.2008.11.127.
7. Oelke M, Bachmann A, Descazeaud A, et al. EAU guidelines on the treatment and follow-up of non-neurogenic male lower urinary tract symptoms including benign prostatic obstruction. Eur Urol 2013;64(1):118–40. http://dx.doi.org/10.1016/j.eururo.2013.03.004.
8. McNicholas TA, Kirby RS, Lepor H. Evaluation and nonsurgical management of benign prostatic hyperplasia. In: Wein AJ, Kavoussi LR, Novick AC, et al, editors. Campbell-Walsh Urology. 10th edition. Philadelphia: Elsevier Saunders; 2012.
9. Lenherr SM, Clemens JQ. Urodynamics: with a focus on appropriate indications. Urol Clin North Am 2013;40(4):545–57. http://dx.doi.org/10.1016/j.ucl.2013.07.001.
10. Chancellor M. Bladder outlet obstruction versus impaired detrusor contractility: the role of outflow. J Urol 1991;145(4):810–2.
11. Oelke M, Baard J, Wijkstra H, et al. Age and bladder outlet obstruction are independently associated with detrusor overactivity in patients with benign prostatic hyperplasia. Eur Urol 2008;54(2):419–26. http://dx.doi.org/10.1016/j.eururo.2008.02.017.
12. Abrams P, Cardozo L, Fall M, et al, Standardisation Subcommittee of the International Continence Society. The standardisation of terminology of lower urinary tract function: report from the Standardisation Sub-committee of the International Continence Society. Neurourol Urodyn 2002;21:167–78.
13. Osman NI, Chapple CR, Abrams P, et al. Detrusor underactivity and the underactive bladder: a new clinical entity? A review of current terminology, definitions, epidemiology, aetiology, and diagnosis. Eur Urol 2013;1–10. http://dx.doi.org/10.1016/j.eururo.2013.10.015.
14. Griffiths D, Hbfner K, Van Mastrigt R, et al. Standardization of terminology of lower urinary tract function: pressure-flow studies of voiding, urethral resistance,

and urethral obstruction. International Continence Society Subcommittee on Standardization of Terminology of Pressure-Flow Studies. Neurourol Urodyn 1997;16:1–18.

15. Mehdizadeh JL, Leach GE. Role of invasive urodynamic testing in benign prostatic hyperplasia and male lower urinary tract symptoms. Urol Clin North Am 2009;36(4):431–41. v. http://dx.doi.org/10.1016/j.ucl.2009.07.002.

16. Nitti VW, Lefkowitz G, Ficazzola M, et al. Lower urinary tract symptoms in young men: videourodynamic findings and correlation with noninvasive measures. J Urol 2002;168(1):135–8. Available at: http://www.ncbi.nlm.nih.gov/pubmed/12050507.

17. Thomas AW, Cannon A, Bartlett E, et al. The natural history of lower urinary tract dysfunction in men: minimum 10-year urodynamic followup of transurethral resection of prostate for bladder outlet obstruction. J Urol 2005;174(5):1887–91. http://dx.doi.org/10.1097/01.ju.0000176740.76061.24.

18. Liao L, Schaefer W. Within-session reproducibility and variability of urethral resistance and detrusor contractility in pressure-flow studies in men with lower urinary tract symptoms. Curr Urol 2009;3(1):19–28. http://dx.doi.org/10.1159/000189677.

19. Tammela TL, Schäfer W, Barrett DM, et al. Repeated pressure-flow studies in the evaluation of bladder outlet obstruction due to benign prostatic enlargement. Finasteride Urodynamics Study Group. Neurourol Urodyn 1999;18(1):17–24. Available at: http://www.ncbi.nlm.nih.gov/pubmed/10090123. Accessed March 4, 2014.

20. Rosier PF, de la Rosette JJ, Koldewijn EL, et al. Variability of pressure-flow analysis parameters in repeated cystometry in patients with benign prostatic hyperplasia. J Urol 1995;153(5):1520–5. Available at: http://www.ncbi.nlm.nih.gov/pubmed/7536260. Accessed March 4, 2014.

21. Wolf JS, Bennett CJ, Dmochowski RR, et al. Best practice policy statement on urologic surgery antimicrobial prophylaxis. J Urol 2008;179(4):1379–90. http://dx.doi.org/10.1016/j.juro.2008.01.068.

22. Scarpero HM, Padmanabhan P, Xue X, et al. Patient perception of videourodynamic testing: a questionnaire based study. J Urol 2005;173(2):555–9. http://dx.doi.org/10.1097/01.ju.0000149968.60938.c0.

23. Ku JH, Kim SW, Kim HH, et al. Patient experience with a urodynamic study: a prospective study in 208 patients. J Urol 2004;171(6):2307–10. http://dx.doi.org/10.1097/01.ju.0000125144.82338.0c.

24. Deber RB, Kraetschmer N, Urowitz S, et al. Do people want to be autonomous patients? Preferred roles in treatment decision-making in several patient populations. Health Expect 2007;10(3):248–58. http://dx.doi.org/10.1111/j.1369-7625.2007.00441.x.

25. Eberth B, Watson V, Ryan M, et al. Does one size fit all? Investigating heterogeneity in men's preferences for benign prostatic hyperplasia treatment using mixed logit analysis. Med Decis Making 2009;29(6):707–15. http://dx.doi.org/10.1177/0272989X09341754.

26. Wills CE, Holmes-Rovner M, Rovner D, et al. Treatment preference patterns during a videotape decision aid for benign prostatic hyperplasia (BPH). Patient Educ Couns 2006;61(1):16–22. http://dx.doi.org/10.1016/j.pec.2005.01.013.

27. Abrams P. In support of pressure-flow studies for evaluating men with lower urinary tract symptoms. Urology 1994;44(2):153–5. Available at: http://www.ncbi.nlm.nih.gov/pubmed/7519378.

28. Tanaka Y, Masumori N, Itoh N, et al. Is the short-term outcome of transurethral resection of the prostate affected by preoperative degree of bladder outlet obstruction, status of detrusor contractility or detrusor overactivity? Int J Urol 2006;13(11):1398–404. http://dx.doi.org/10.1111/j.1442-2042.2006.01589.x.

29. Machino R, Kakizaki H, Ameda K, et al. Detrusor instability with equivocal obstruction: a predictor of unfavorable symptomatic outcomes after transurethral prostatectomy. Neurourol Urodyn 2002;21(5):444–9. http://dx.doi.org/10.1002/nau.10057.

30. Van Venrooij GE, van Melick HH, Boon TA. Comparison of outcomes of transurethral prostate resection in urodynamically obstructed versus selected urodynamically unobstructed or equivocal men. Urol 2003;62(4):672–6. http://dx.doi.org/10.1016/S0090-4295(03)00511-9.

31. DiSantostefano R, Biddle A, Lavelle J. An evaluation of the economic costs and patient-related consequences of treatments for benign prostatic hyperplasia. Br J Urol 2006;97:1007–16. http://dx.doi.org/10.1111/j.1464-410X.2006.06089.x.

Urodynamics in Pelvic Organ Prolapse
When Are They Helpful and How Do We Use Them?

Katie N. Ballert, MD

KEYWORDS

- Pelvic organ prolapse • Urodynamics • Occult stress urinary incontinence • Stress testing
- Detrusor overactivity

KEY POINTS

- The utility of urodynamics in women with pelvic organ prolapse (POP) is still being elucidated.
- Urodynamics can be used to identify stress incontinence on prolapse reduction (occult stress urinary incontinence [SUI]) in patients with POP.
- In patients who are clinically continent, urodynamics may be useful if patients and physicians are amenable to selective management of the urethra at the time of POP repair.
- The usefulness of urodynamics seems limited in patients with POP and overactive bladder (OAB) symptoms.
- The decision to perform preoperative urodynamics should be made on an individual basis and with a clear understanding of how the results will have an impact on patient counseling or treatment.

INTRODUCTION

POP is a common clinical condition that affects millions of women. There is an estimated 11.1% lifetime risk that a woman will undergo surgery for POP or incontinence by 80 years of age, with a 30% reoperation rate.[1] POP and urinary incontinence have a significant impact on quality of life[2] and health care costs.[3] The number of patients seeking treatment of POP and urinary incontinence is predicted to increase dramatically over the next several years. The incidence of POP and urinary incontinence has been found to increase with advanced age.[1] According to United Nations World Population Ageing data, the number of persons age 60 or older has surpassed 700 million and it is projected that by 2050 2 billion persons 60 years or older will be alive.[4] Luber and colleagues[5] note that women over the age of 60 are more likely to seek medical care for pelvic floor disorders and predict a 45% increase in the demand for treatment of pelvic floor disorders including POP over the next 30 years.

Urodynamics (specifically, filling cystometrogram and pressure flow urodynamics) has become a standard part of the evaluation of patients with POP and/or urinary incontinence for many providers. The routine use of preoperative urodynamics in all patients, however, has been under increasing amounts of scrutiny as the medical community seeks to practice evidence-based medicine. POP can be associated with various lower urinary tract symptoms, including storage symptoms, urinary incontinence and voiding symptoms; however, it is often unclear how these symptoms will correlate with urodynamic findings. It is also unclear if urodynamic findings will

Division of Urology, Department of Surgery, University of Kentucky, 800 Rose Street, MS 269, Lexington, KY 40536-0298, USA
E-mail address: kba224@uky.edu

Urol Clin N Am 41 (2014) 409–417
http://dx.doi.org/10.1016/j.ucl.2014.04.001
0094-0143/14/$ – see front matter © 2014 Elsevier Inc. All rights reserved.

urologic.theclinics.com

correlate with postoperative outcomes or how the data should have an impact on patient counseling and surgical planning.

EVALUATION FOR STRESS INCONTINENCE ON PROLAPSE REDUCTION (OCCULT STRESS URINARY INCONTINENCE)

Stress incontinence on prolapse reduction, also known as occult SUI or latent stress incontinence, is SUI that occurs in women with POP only after the prolapse is reduced. It is thought related to kinking of the urethra[6] that is relieved with prolapse reduction. Prolapse reduction has been reported to unmask SUI on prolapse reduction in 36% to 80% of clinically continent women with severe POP.[6–8] In a review of the records of 24 continent women with stage 3 or 4 prolapse, Chaikin and colleagues[7] found that 14 (58%) had demonstrable SUI on urodynamic testing with a pessary in place. Gordon and colleagues[9] evaluated 45 clinically continent women with stage 3 POP, of whom 30 (67%) demonstrated SUI after repositioning the prolapse with a ring pessary during preoperative urodynamic evaluation. Ghoniem and colleagues[10] found that in 11 of 16 (69%) continent women with large cystoceles, SUI was noted on evaluation after prolapse reduction with vaginal packing.

In addition, POP repair was previously shown to result in postoperative SUI in 11% to 22% of clinically continent women.[11,12] Stanton and colleagues[11] reported an 11% rate of postoperative SUI within 3 months in a group of patients undergoing anterior colporrhaphy with or without vaginal hysterectomy. Borstad and Rud[12] found that 22% of clinically continent women undergoing a Manchester procedure for POP had postoperative SUI.

Several studies have documented the use of urodynamics to demonstrate stress incontinence on prolapse reduction in women with POP; however, its impact on postoperative outcomes remains highly debated. Most investigators agree that in patients with POP and symptomatic SUI, a simultaneous anti-incontinence procedure should be performed. Urodynamics is often used to evaluate patients with POP who do not have clinical SUI in an effort to identify those patients who are at risk for developing postoperative SUI and thus may benefit from simultaneous anti-incontinence procedure. The question remains, however: Can preoperative urodynamics be relied on to accurately predict those patients who will develop postoperative SUI without a simultaneous anti-incontinence procedure? And, should those patients without SUI demonstrated on urodynamics with reduction of prolapse be recommended to have POP repair alone?

The author and colleagues previously evaluated a urodynamic protocol used for managing the urethra at the time of transvaginal POP repair,[13] looking at 105 patients with stages 2–4 POP in which a simultaneous midurethral synthetic sling was performed at the time of transvaginal POP repair if urodynamic SUI or SUI on prolapse reduction was demonstrated. If there was no demonstrable SUI on urodynamics with or without prolapse reduction, then a sling was not performed. Using this protocol, when a midurethral synthetic sling was placed, the risk of intervention due to obstruction (8.5%) was found essentially equal to the risk of subsequent intervention for SUI (8.3%) when no clinical, urodynamic, or SUI on prolapse reduction was present and no sling was placed. These data suggest that urodynamics may identify a subset of patients who may not need a prophylactic anti-incontinence procedure at the time of transvaginal POP repair. Also, in patients who reported clinical SUI but did not demonstrate SUI on urodynamic with or without reduction of prolapse, and thus did not have a simultaneous sling, the risk of postoperative intervention for SUI was 30%. It could be argued that based on the 30% risk of repeat surgery, a simultaneous sling should be performed in all patients with clinical SUI regardless of urodynamic findings indicating that preoperative urodynamics may not be necessary in these patients. Conversely, the urodynamic results could be used to counsel the small subset of patients with clinical SUI but no urodynamic SUI or SUI on prolapse reduction that there is a 70% chance that they would not require a second surgery.

In another study, Chermansky and colleagues[14] evaluated postoperative incontinence and patient satisfaction using selective management of the urethra at the time of POP repair. They evaluated 42 patients with advanced apical and/or anterior compartment POP. Patients with clinical, occult, or urodynamic SUI were treated with a simultaneous sling procedure. Those without clinical or demonstrable SUI were treated with POP repair alone: 30 patients completed all of the postoperative questionnaires (Urogenital Distress Inventory [UDI-6], Patient Global Impression of Improvement [PGI-I], and Medical, Epidemiological, and Social Aspects of Aging [MESA]); 14 of the patients underwent only POP repair; and 16 patients had a POP repair with sling. There was no statistically significant difference in questionnaire results between those patients who underwent POP repair alone and those who had a simultaneous sling procedure. The mean of both groups reported their condition as "much better" on the PGI-I questionnaire. Only 1 patient in the POP repair–only group returned with postoperative SUI and underwent a subsequent sling procedure. The investigators also evaluated the cost variance between the 2 groups and found an estimated total cost savings of $55,804 using selective management.

Elser and colleagues[15] evaluated the use of preoperative urodynamics to determine the need for an anti-incontinence procedure at the time of abdominal sacrocolpopexy. They retrospectively reviewed 463 patients who underwent abdominal sacrocolpopexy; 204 patients had SUI on preoperative urodynamics either with or without prolapse reduction and 237 patients had no SUI. All of the patients with preoperative SUI underwent a simultaneous anti-incontinence procedure; 157 patients (77%) underwent a midurethral synthetic sling (either retropubic or transobturator) and 47 patients (23%) underwent Burch urethropexy. Charts were available for review on 441 patients. At 6 weeks postoperatively, 178 (87.3%) of the patients who had SUI and underwent an anti-incontinence procedure and 220 (92.8%) of the patients without preoperative SUI, and thus no anti-incontinence procedure, reported no incontinence. The authors concluded that urodynamics is useful in determining the need for an anti-incontinence procedure at the time of abdominal sacrocolpopexy and recommended that patients without preoperative SUI (including SUI with reduction of prolapse) not undergo simultaneous anti-incontinence surgery.

In addition to these studies, several other small studies have suggested that clinically continent patients without urodynamic SUI with reduction of prolapse are unlikely to develop postoperative SUI after POP repair.[7,16,17] Some also demonstrate a high rate of postoperative SUI in patients with SUI on prolapse reduction who did not undergo a simultaneous anti-incontinence procedure.[16,17]

In a study by Chaikin and colleagues,[7] 24 women without clinical symptoms of SUI were evaluated; 14 patients were found to have SUI on prolapse reduction during urodynamic evaluation and underwent an autologous fascia sling. Of the 10 patients who did not have a sling, none developed postoperative SUI at an average of almost 4 years' follow-up. Another small retrospective study by Araki and colleagues[16] evaluated the utility of preoperative urodynamics to predict postoperative urinary symptoms. They evaluated records of 87 patients who underwent surgery for POP. Of the 22 patients with SUI on prolapse reduction, 13 did not undergo simultaneous transobturator midurethral synthetic sling. Of those 13 patients, 62% developed symptomatic postoperative SUI; 49 patients did not demonstrate SUI on prolapse reduction on preoperative urodynamics; and only 2 (4%) developed postoperative SUI.

Liang and colleagues[17] reported on 79 patients with severe POP but without clinical SUI; 30 patients did not demonstrate SUI on prolapse reduction on preoperative urodynamics and underwent POP repair alone. None of the 30 patients developed SUI postoperatively. Furthermore, in the 49 patients who had SUI on prolapse reduction on preoperative urodynamics, POP repair alone was performed in 17 patients and simultaneous tension-free vaginal tape (TVT) was performed in 32 patients. The investigators found that patients with SUI on prolapse reduction who underwent POP repair alone had a significantly higher rate of subjective and objective SUI compared with patients who underwent simultaneous TVT placement (64.7% and 53% vs 10% and 0%, respectively). In the author and colleagues' study[13] (discussed previously), 22 of 24 women (91.7%) without symptomatic or SUI on prolapse reduction did not require further intervention for SUI after POP repair.

There are also studies that question the utility of stress testing during urodynamics in women with prolapse.[18–20] Recently, the Outcomes Following Vaginal Prolapse Repair and Mid Urethral Sling (OPUS) Trial found that a prophylactic midurethral synthetic sling performed at the time of transvaginal POP repair resulted in lower rates of urinary incontinence at 3 and 12 months postoperatively regardless of preoperative prolapse reduction stress testing.[18] In this study Wei and colleagues[18] evaluated 337 women with anterior prolapse (stage 2 or higher) without symptoms of SUI who were planning to undergo transvaginal POP repair. Evaluation included a preoperative prolapse reduction stress test (at a bladder volume of 300 mL with the prolapse reduced with 1 or 2 large swabs) but did not include preoperative urodynamic evaluation. Women were randomly assigned to undergo simultaneous midurethral synthetic sling or sham incisions during the POP repair. All the slings placed were performed in a retropubic fashion (Gynecare TVT, Ethicon, Bridgewater, NJ, USA); however, the transvaginal procedures performed to address the POP varied.

Of the randomized patients, 327 (97%) completed 1-year follow-up. At 3 months' follow-up, 23.6% who had a sling and 49.4% of patients in the sham group had postoperative SUI. At 12 months, urinary incontinence (allowing for subsequent treatment) was present in 27.3% and 43.0%, respectively. The number needed to treat with a sling to prevent 1 case of urinary incontinence at 1 year was 6.3. Preoperatively, 33.5% of women had a positive prolapse reduction stress test. At 3 months, 29.6% of the sling group versus 71.9% of the sham group had urinary incontinence, indicating that women with a positive stress test preoperatively received more benefit from a sling than those with a negative test. This difference was not statistically significant at 12 months, however. During the first year postoperatively, 1 woman (0.6%) in the sling group underwent surgery for urinary incontinence and 4 (2.4%) underwent surgery for voiding dysfunction. Adverse events, including bladder perforation, major bleeding complications, and incomplete bladder emptying in the first 6 weeks after surgery, were also all more common in the sling group than in the sham group.

Visco and colleagues[19] questioned the utility of stress testing specifically during urodynamics in women with prolapse based on findings from the Colpopexy and Urinary Reduction Efforts (CARE) trial. The CARE trial found that a significant number of patients who did not leak during preoperative testing developed postoperative SUI. In the trial, 322 patients undergoing abdominal sacrocolpopexy for stages II–IV POP were randomized to concomitant Burch colposuspension (157 patients) or to the control group (165 patients). Of the women in each group, 36% had SUI on prolapse reduction on preoperative urodynamics. In the control group (no Burch), postoperative SUI occurred in 38% with a negative stress reduction test.

The CARE trial has been cited as level 1 evidence that a Burch colposuspension should routinely be performed at the time of abdominal sacrocolpopexy.[20] At 3 months postoperatively, 23.6% of the women who underwent Burch colposuspension versus 44.1% of controls met at least 1 criterion for SUI. Furthermore, Burch colposuspension decreased SUI postoperatively even in the patients who did not have SUI on prolapse reduction preoperatively (20.8% vs 38.2%). Togami and colleagues[21] pointed out, however, that in the CARE trial, 62% of patients did not leak after abdominal sacrocolpopexy alone, highlighting that greater than 50% of patients would be overtreated. They also noted that Burch colposuspension only resulted in an 18% reduction in postoperative SUI.

The CARE trial found that women who demonstrated preoperative urodynamic SUI on prolapse reduction were more likely to have postoperative SUI regardless of whether they underwent a simultaneous Burch procedure. In the control group, 58% percent of patients with a positive stress reduction test developed postoperative SUI compared with 38% of those with a negative stress reduction test. In the group who underwent simultaneous Burch, 32% with a positive stress test experienced postoperative SUI compared with 21% of patients with a negative test. The

investigators acknowledged that this information could be used for preoperative counseling but questioned whether it would have an impact on patient management.[19]

METHODS OF PROLAPSE REDUCTION

Some investigators have criticized the ability of preoperative testing to reproduce the postoperative anatomic urethral positioning and thus its ability to accurately identify patients who will develop SUI.[22,23] Currently, there is no standardized method of prolapse reduction used to test for SUI on prolapse reduction. In the CARE trial, rates of detection of SUI on prolapse reduction varied based on the method of prolapse reduction.[19] Use of a pessary resulted in the lowest rates at 6% and the speculum was the highest at 30%. They also evaluated manual reduction (16%), reduction with a swab (20%), and reduction with ring forceps (21%). The sensitivity of the reduction tests ranged from 5% to 39% and the specificity from 74% to 96%. During reduction testing, adequately reducing the prolapse while avoiding artificial obstruction of the urethra or overcorrection of the urethrovesical junction must be attempted. Reproducibility of the reduction maneuvers has also been shown to vary based on the characteristics of the prolapse.[24] Patients who have complete vault eversion may require more aggressive maneuvers to reduce the prolapse. This may lead to excessive flattening of the posterior urethrovaginal angle and a false-positive stress test.[24]

EVALUATION OF CONCOMITANT STORAGE SYMPTOMS

Frequency, urgency, and urinary urgency incontinence (UUI) are reported to occur in up to 86% of patients with POP.[2,25,26] Furthermore, surgical treatment of POP has been reported to improve frequency and UUI in 31% to 76% and 49% to 82% of patients, respectively.[27–29] The utility of urodynamics to predict persistent postoperative storage symptoms after POP repair is, however, poorly defined.

In the retrospective study by Araki and colleagues,[16] detrusor overactivity was demonstrated in 31% of patients with urinary urgency. After POP repair, urgency persisted in 87% (13/15) of patients who demonstrated detrusor overactivity on preoperative urodynamics. It resolved in 70% (23/33) of patients who did not demonstrate detrusor overactivity preoperatively.[16] In another study, Fletcher and colleagues[27] retrospectively evaluated 88 patients who underwent an anterior vaginal prolapse repair. Evaluation included preoperative and postoperative UDI-6 scores for frequency and UUI as well as preoperative urodynamics. Detrusor overactivity was demonstrated in 20 (19%) of the patients preoperatively. They found that 31% of patients had improvement in urinary frequency and 49% had improvement in UUI postoperatively, but preoperative detrusor overactivity did not correlate with resolution or persistence of symptoms. The only variable that emerged as an independent risk factor for persistent UUI postoperatively was higher preoperative detrusor pressure at maximum flow. They suggested that prolapse-induced obstruction may contribute to alterations in detrusor function that led to persistent OAB symptoms.

Wolter and colleagues[30] retrospectively reviewed 111 patients who underwent anterior POP repair and sling procedure. Preoperatively, 54% presented with symptoms of mixed urinary incontinence, 25% SUI, and 9% UUI. The remaining 12% were asymptomatic but demonstrated SUI on prolapse reduction. The patients with UUI also had SUI on prolapse reduction; 35 patients (31.5%) had detrusor overactivity on preoperative urodynamics. The rate of urgency/UUI decreased from 63% (70/111) preoperatively to 30% (33/111) postoperatively. Preoperative detrusor overactivity was not predictive, however, of persistent postoperative urge-related symptoms. The rate of urgency/frequency was 28.6% (10/35) in the patients with preoperative detrusor overactivity and 30.3% (23/76) in the patients without detrusor overactivity on preoperative urodynamics.

It is not surprising that preoperative detrusor overactivity has not been consistently shown to correlate with postoperative symptom persistence or resolution. It is well known that many patients with frequency, urgency, and UUI do not demonstrate detrusor overactivity on urodynamics,[31] whereas other patients who do not have lower urinary tract symptoms demonstrate detrusor overactivity.[32] Foster and colleagues[29] previously noted a lack of correlation between OAB symptoms and demonstrable urodynamic detrusor overactivity. They prospectively evaluated 65 elderly women undergoing transvaginal surgery for advanced POP. Detrusor overactivity was documented on preoperative urodynamics in 25% of the patients, but preoperative urodynamic parameters did not correlate with the presence or absence of OAB symptoms. Only 2 (7%) patients with UUI had demonstrable detrusor overactivity on preoperative urodynamics. They also demonstrated significant improvement in OAB symptoms after POP repair. At 12 months, they found that urgency, frequency, and UUI resolved in 76%, 54.6%, and 75% of patients, respectively.

It seems that urodynamic findings may be of limited value for preoperative counseling in patients with POP and OAB. They are also unlikely to have an impact on surgical planning in these patients. Urodynamics should be performed in patients with neurologic disease or risk factors for impaired bladder compliance, however, especially if a simultaneous anti-incontinence procedure is considered at the time of POP repair. Increasing outlet resistance in the face of impaired compliance could be detrimental to renal function.

EVALUATION OF VOIDING SYMPTOMS OR ELEVATED POSTVOID RESIDUAL

Bladder outlet obstruction is a common urodynamic finding among women with advanced POP.[33,34] Approximately 21% of women with stage 2 POP and 33% of those with stage 3 or 4 POP report difficulty with bladder emptying.[35] These symptoms may improve after surgical correction of the prolapse due to resolution of the obstruction.[34] It has also been suggested that bladder outlet obstruction may contribute to OAB symptoms in women with advanced POP.[27,36]

The American Urological Association (AUA)/Society for Urodynamics and Female Urology (SUFU) guideline on urodynamic studies in adults states that urodynamics with POP reduction may be used to assess for detrusor dysfunction in women with associated lower urinary tract symptoms. The investigators suggested that urodynamics with POP reduction may help determine if elevated postvoid residual urine (PVR) is due to detrusor underactivity or outlet obstruction or a combination of the two.[37] Some investigators have suggested factoring elevated PVR or detrusor underactivity into protocols that determine the need for simultaneous anti-incontinence procedure at the time of POP repair.[21,38] Many investigators suggest avoiding simultaneous sling placement in patients at risk for voiding disorders, but this patient population has not been well defined.[13,21,38] Furthermore, few studies have actually examined the utility of urodynamics to predict postoperative voiding dysfunction after POP with or without simultaneous anti-incontinence procedure.

Romanzi and colleagues[34] prospectively evaluated 60 women with grades 1 to 4 POP to determine if POP causes obstruction that can be relieved by reduction with a pessary. They found that 70% of women with grades 3 and 4 prolapse (Baden-Walker) had urodynamic bladder outlet obstruction compared with only 3% of those with grades 1 and 2 POP. They defined bladder outlet obstruction as maximum detrusor pressure at a maximum flow of greater than 25 cm H_2O with maximum flow less than 15 mL/s. They also found that 94% of those women with grade 3 or 4 POP and bladder outlet obstruction had normal free uroflowmetry after prolapse reduction with a ring pessary. Furthermore, 13% of women met their criteria for impaired detrusor contractility, which they defined as maximum detrusor pressure less than 15 cm H_2O, with maximum flow less than 15 mL/s. The study did not comment, however, on treatment or postoperative outcomes for these patients.

Fletcher and colleagues[27] also looked at voiding difficulty in their retrospective study of 88 women who underwent anterior vaginal wall POP repair. Preoperatively, 30 (29%) patients reported difficulty emptying. Operative management resulted in improvement in the voiding symptoms in 74% of those patients. Patients with improvement in difficulty emptying had significantly higher preoperative PVR volumes than those without improvement (129 mL vs 31 mL). Improvement was not related to higher cystocele grade but was correlated with older age.

Mueller and colleagues[39] evaluated 31 women with advanced POP undergoing urodynamics and found that there was no statistically significant difference in maximum cystometric capacity, voided volume, maximal flow, or detrusor pressure at maximal flow with or without prolapse reduction. The only significant difference was a decrease in maximum urethral closure pressure with prolapse reduction. Despite no difference in the voiding parameters, when they applied the criteria of bladder outlet obstruction used by Romanzi and colleagues[34] to their patient population, 40% of patients met the criteria for obstruction when the prolapse was not reduced, whereas only 17% met the criteria with reduction. As in Romanzi and colleagues' study, there was no mention of treatment or postoperative outcomes in the study.

Finally, there are several studies evaluating the ability of preoperative urodynamics to identify patients at risk for voiding dysfunction after anti-incontinence procedures.[40–43] These studies provide conflicting data regarding the utility of urodynamics. Some of the studies included patients undergoing simultaneous prolapse repair, but they were not designed to specifically evaluate patients with preoperative voiding symptoms or elevated PVR.

OTHER OPTIONS FOR PREOPERATIVE TESTING IN PATIENTS WITH POP

The AUA/SUFU guideline states that stress testing should be performed with reduction of the POP in women with high-grade POP without the symptoms of SUI.[37] If SUI on prolapse reduction is the only thing looked for, however, then a simple stress test with the prolapse reduced can be performed and urodynamics may be avoided in patients with a positive result. Another option is a trial of pessary. This allows for evaluation during patients' normal daily activities. This relies on patients agreeing to a trial of pessary and having a successful fitting. Prior studies have reported successful pessary fitting trial rates in 63% to 74% of patients.[44–47] Rates vary depending on the definition used. Handa and Jones[46] retrospectively evaluated 56 consecutive women treated with a pessary for symptomatic POP. They initially used ring pessaries for fitting and, if needed, a donut pessary was used; 64% or women had a successful fitting; 5 women (9%) failed fitting at the first visit; and an additional 15 women (27%) discontinued use within 3 months.[46] Clemons and colleagues[44] reported on 100 consecutive women with POP who underwent pessary fitting; 73 had a successful 2-week trial, and, among the women without baseline SUI, 21% developed SUI on prolapse reduction.

Chughtai and colleagues[47] evaluated the use of an ambulatory pessary trial to evaluate for SUI on prolapse reduction in women undergoing surgical repair of POP. They evaluated patients with preoperative urodynamics with and without prolapse reduction and offered them a home pessary trial. Of the 41 women who accepted the pessary trial, 26 (63.4%) were able to retain the pessary for at least 1 week; 10 of the 26 women (38%) did not have SUI (clinical, on physical examination, during urodynamic testing, or during the pessary trial) and underwent POP repair alone. None of these women developed postoperative SUI: 16 (61%) demonstrated SUI on prolapse reduction; 3 of these (19%) had negative stress testing during video urodynamics and were identified only by the pessary trial. They also found that the pessary test accurately predicted persistent urgency, frequency, and voiding difficulty. They specifically recommended a home pessary trial for women with severe POP and no evidence of SUI during urodynamics; however, physicians could also consider offering a home pessary test instead of urodynamics.

Another option is provocative stress testing with a pessary in place. Reena and colleagues[48] used a pessary test to evaluate for SUI on prolapse reduction in 88 continent women. All participants were fitted with a pessary and given pyridium. They then underwent a regimen of provocative exercises (stair climbing, standing from a sitting position, coughing, and stooping) and their pad was examined for orange discoloration. Participants subsequently underwent vaginal hysterectomy and POP repair without a simultaneous anti-incontinence procedure; 10 women were lost to follow-up. Of the remaining 78 women, 68% had a positive test and, of these, 64.2% developed postoperative SUI at 6 weeks' follow-up; 25 women did not demonstrate SUI on prolapse reduction preoperatively and all remained continent at 6 weeks.

SUMMARY

The utility of urodynamics in patients with POP is still being elucidated. It is not a requirement for all patients planning surgical repair. The need for urodynamics prior to POP repair should be determined for each individual patient. Prior to performance of urodynamics, physicians should consider how the results will impact on preoperative patient counseling or surgical planning.

The usefulness of urodynamics seems limited in patients with POP and OAB symptoms as well as in those with straightforward clinical SUI. In patients who are clinically continent, however, urodynamics may be useful if patient and physician are amenable to selective management of the urethra at the time of POP repair. This decision can be made only after counseling a patient and determining preference regarding a simultaneous prophylactic anti-incontinence procedure versus the risk of requiring a second procedure. The potential complications of anti-incontinence procedures (de novo OAB, bladder outlet obstruction, and mesh-related complications if a synthetic sling is performed) must also be considered. Complications rates after sling procedures are higher in women with high-stage POP[49] and patients should be aware of this.

REFERENCES

1. Olsen AL, Smith VJ, Bergstrom JO, et al. Epidemiology of surgically managed pelvic organ prolapse and urinary incontinence. Obstet Gynecol 1997;89(4):501–6.
2. Digesu GA, Chaliha C, Salvatore S, et al. The relationship of vaginal prolapse severity to symptoms and quality of life. BJOG 2005;112(7):971–6.
3. Cheon C, Maher C. Economics of pelvic organ prolapse surgery. Int Urogynecol J 2013;24(11):1873–6.
4. United Nations. World Population Ageing. 2009. Available at: www.un.org/esa/population/publications/WPA2009. Accessed December 13, 2013.
5. Luber KM, Boero S, Choe JY. The demographics of pelvic floor disorders: current observations and future projections. Am J Obstet Gynecol 2001;184(7):1496–501 [discussion: 1501–3].
6. Richardson DA, Bent AE, Ostergard DR. The effect of uterovaginal prolapse on urethrovesical pressure dynamics. Am J Obstet Gynecol 1983;146(8):901–5.
7. Chaikin DC, Groutz A, Blaivas JG. Predicting the need for anti-incontinence surgery in continent women undergoing repair of severe urogenital prolapse. J Urol 2000;163(2):531–4.
8. Bergman A, Koonings PP, Ballard CA. Predicting postoperative urinary incontinence development in women undergoing operation for genitourinary prolapse. Am J Obstet Gynecol 1988;158(5):1171–5.
9. Gordon D, Groutz A, Wolman I, et al. Development of postoperative urinary stress incontinence in clinically continent patients undergoing prophylactic Kelly plication during genitourinary prolapse repair. Neurourol Urodyn 1999;18(3):193–7 [discussion: 197–8].
10. Ghoniem GM, Walters F, Lewis V. The value of the vaginal pack test in large cystoceles. J Urol 1994;152(3):931–4.
11. Stanton SL, Hilton P, Norton C, et al. Clinical and urodynamic effects of anterior colporrhaphy and vaginal hysterectomy for prolapse with and without incontinence. Br J Obstet Gynaecol 1982;89(6):459–63.
12. Borstad E, Rud T. The risk of developing urinary stress-incontinence after vaginal repair in continent women. A clinical and urodynamic follow-up study. Acta Obstet Gynecol Scand 1989;68(6):545–9.
13. Ballert KN, Biggs GY, Isenalumhe A Jr, et al. Managing the urethra at transvaginal pelvic organ prolapse repair: a urodynamic approach. J Urol 2009;181(2):679–84.
14. Chermansky CJ, Krlin RM, Winters JC. Selective management of the urethra at time of pelvic organ prolapse repair: an assessment of postoperative incontinence and patient satisfaction. J Urol 2012;187(6):2144–8.
15. Elser DM, Moen MD, Stanford EJ, et al. Abdominal sacrocolpopexy and urinary incontinence: surgical planning based on urodynamics. Am J Obstet Gynecol 2010;202(4):375.e1–5.
16. Araki I, Haneda Y, Mikami Y, et al. Incontinence and detrusor dysfunction associated with pelvic organ prolapse: clinical value of preoperative urodynamic evaluation. Int Urogynecol J Pelvic Floor Dysfunct 2009;20(11):1301–6.
17. Liang CC, Chang YL, Chang SD, et al. Pessary test to predict postoperative urinary incontinence in women undergoing hysterectomy for prolapse. Obstet Gynecol 2004;104(4):795–800.
18. Wei JT, Nygaard I, Richter HE, et al. A midurethral sling to reduce incontinence after vaginal prolapse repair. N Engl J Med 2012;366(25):2358–67.

19. Visco AG, Brubaker L, Nygaard I, et al. The role of preoperative urodynamic testing in stress-continent women undergoing sacrocolpopexy: the Colpopexy and Urinary Reduction Efforts (CARE) randomized surgical trial. Int Urogynecol J Pelvic Floor Dysfunct 2008;19(5):607–14.

20. Brubaker L, Cundiff GW, Fine P, et al. Abdominal sacrocolpopexy with Burch colposuspension to reduce urinary stress incontinence. N Engl J Med 2006;354(15):1557–66.

21. Togami JM, Chow D, Winters JC. To sling or not to sling at the time of anterior vaginal compartment repair. Curr Opin Urol 2010;20(4):269–74.

22. Twiss C, Triaca V, Raz S. Re: Reevaluating occult stress incontinence. Eur Urol 2007;51(3):850–1.

23. Roovers JP, Oelke M. Clinical relevance of urodynamic investigation tests prior to surgical correction of genital prolapse: a literature review. Int Urogynecol J Pelvic Floor Dysfunct 2007;18(4): 455–60.

24. Karram MM. What is the optimal anti-incontinence procedure in women with advanced prolapse and 'potential' stress incontinence? Int Urogynecol J Pelvic Floor Dysfunct 1999;10(1):1–2.

25. Bradley CS, Nygaard IE. Vaginal wall descensus and pelvic floor symptoms in older women. Obstet Gynecol 2005;106(4):759–66.

26. Gutman RE, Ford DE, Quiroz LH, et al. Is there a pelvic organ prolapse threshold that predicts pelvic floor symptoms? Am J Obstet Gynecol 2008; 199(6):683.e1–7.

27. Fletcher SG, Haverkorn RM, Yan J, et al. Demographic and urodynamic factors associated with persistent OAB after anterior compartment prolapse repair. Neurourol Urodyn 2010;29(8):1414–8.

28. Digesu GA, Salvatore S, Chaliha C, et al. Do overactive bladder symptoms improve after repair of anterior vaginal wall prolapse? Int Urogynecol J Pelvic Floor Dysfunct 2007;18(12):1439–43.

29. Foster RT Sr, Barber MD, Parasio MF, et al. A prospective assessment of overactive bladder symptoms in a cohort of elderly women who underwent transvaginal surgery for advanced pelvic organ prolapse. Am J Obstet Gynecol 2007;197(1): 82.e1–4.

30. Wolter CE, Kaufman MR, Duffy JW, et al. Mixed incontinence and cystocele: postoperative urge symptoms are not predicted by preoperative urodynamics. Int Urogynecol J 2011;22(3):321–5.

31. Rosenzweig BA, Pushkin S, Blumenfeld D, et al. Prevalence of abnormal urodynamic test results in continent women with severe genitourinary prolapse. Obstet Gynecol 1992;79(4):539–42.

32. van Waalwijk van Doorn ES, Remmers A, Janknegt RA. Conventional and extramural ambulatory urodynamic testing of the lower urinary tract in female volunteers. J Urol 1992;147(5):1319–25 [discussion: 1326].

33. Groutz A, Blaivas JG, Chaikin DC. Bladder outlet obstruction in women: definition and characteristics. Neurourol Urodyn 2000;19(3):213–20.

34. Romanzi LJ, Chaikin DC, Blaivas JG. The effect of genital prolapse on voiding. J Urol 1999;161(2): 581–6.

35. Slieker-ten Hove MC, Pool-Goudzwaard AL, Eijkemans MJ, et al. The prevalence of pelvic organ prolapse symptoms and signs and their relation with bladder and bowel disorders in a general female population. Int Urogynecol J Pelvic Floor Dysfunct 2009;20(9):1037–45.

36. Basu M, Duckett J. Effect of prolapse repair on voiding and the relationship to overactive bladder and detrusor overactivity. Int Urogynecol J Pelvic Floor Dysfunct 2009;20(5):499–504.

37. Winters JC, Dmochowski RR, Goldman HB, et al. Urodynamic studies in adults: AUA/SUFU guideline. J Urol 2012;188(Suppl 6):2464–72.

38. Fatton B. Is there any evidence to advocate SUI prevention in continent women undergoing prolapse repair? An overview. Int Urogynecol J Pelvic Floor Dysfunct 2009;20(2):235–45.

39. Mueller ER, Kenton K, Mahajan S, et al. Urodynamic prolapse reduction alters urethral pressure but not filling or pressure flow parameters. J Urol 2007; 177(2):600–3.

40. Miller EA, Amundsen CL, Toh KL, et al. Preoperative urodynamic evaluation may predict voiding dysfunction in women undergoing pubovaginal sling. J Urol 2003;169(6):2234–7.

41. Lemack GE, Krauss S, Litman H, et al. Normal preoperative urodynamic testing does not predict voiding dysfunction after Burch colposuspension versus pubovaginal sling. J Urol 2008;180(5): 2076–80.

42. Wang KH, Wang KH, Neimark M, et al. Voiding dysfunction following TVT procedure. Int Urogynecol J Pelvic Floor Dysfunct 2002;13(6):353–7 [discussion: 358].

43. Pham KN, Topp N, Guralnick ML, et al. Preoperative Valsalva voiding increases the risk of urinary retention after midurethral sling placement. Int Urogynecol J 2010;21(10):1243–6.

44. Clemons JL, Aguilar VC, Tillinghast TA, et al. Patient satisfaction and changes in prolapse and urinary symptoms in women who were fitted successfully with a pessary for pelvic organ prolapse. Am J Obstet Gynecol 2004;190(4):1025–9.

45. Clemons JL, Aguilar VC, Tillinghast TA, et al. Risk factors associated with an unsuccessful pessary fitting trial in women with pelvic organ prolapse. Am J Obstet Gynecol 2004;190(2): 345–50.

46. Handa VL, Jones M. Do pessaries prevent the progression of pelvic organ prolapse? Int Urogynecol J Pelvic Floor Dysfunct 2002;13:349–52.

47. Chughtai B, Spettel S, Kurman J, et al. Ambulatory pessary trial unmasks occult stress urinary incontinence. Obstet Gynecol Int 2012;2012:392027.

48. Reena C, Kekre AN, Kekre N. Occult stress incontinence in women with pelvic organ prolapse. Int J Gynaecol Obstet 2007;97(1):31–4.

49. Anger JT, Litwin MS, Wang Q, et al. The effect of concomitant prolapse repair on sling outcomes. J Urol 2008;180(3):1003–6.

Urodynamics for Postprostatectomy Incontinence
When Are They Helpful and How Do We Use Them?

Ying H. Jura, MD*, Craig V. Comiter, MD

KEYWORDS

- Postprostatectomy incontinence • Urodynamics • Stress urinary incontinence
- Detrusor underacitivity • Detrusor overactivity • Low bladder compliance
- Artificial urinary sphincter • Male sling

KEY POINTS

- Urodynamics is indicated for the evaluation of postprostatectomy incontinence (PPI) unless an artificial urinary sphincter (AUS) placement is the preferred option, as in cases of severe incontinence, prior radiation, or previous male sling or AUS placement—when male sling is unlikely to achieve efficacy.
- Urodynamics should be performed only when there is a question it can answer that would affect treatment choice or outcome.
- Urodynamic findings of detrusor underactivity, overactivity, and reduced compliance are important considerations in deciding how best to treat postprostatectomy incontinence.

INTRODUCTION

Approximately 70% of men 2 years after radical prostatectomy suffer some degree of PPI and 1% to 5% of these patients ultimately seek surgical management of their incontinence after radical prostatectomy.[1–4] The rate of incontinence after surgery for benign prostatic hyperplasia (BPH) is much lower, approximately 2%.[5] Although stress urinary incontinence (SUI) is the most common cause of PPI, urgency incontinence, mixed incontinence, and overflow incontinence must also be considered. Furthermore, 50% to 70% of men with postprostatectomy SUI have some form of concurrent bladder dysfunction (overactivity, underactivity, or decreased bladder compliance).[6–8] Urodynamic testing is an important part of the PPI evaluation when the pathophysiology of PPI is unclear or if a patient is planning to undergo invasive anti-incontinence surgery. Urodynamics can uncover concurrent bladder dysfunction (such as detrusor underactivity, overactivity, or poor compliance) and quantify the degree of bladder neck and proximal urethral mobility as well as the degree of intrinsic sphincter deficiency (ISD). These findings may be helpful in providing prognostic information for the patient and for selecting the most appropriate treatment options.

Department of Urology, Stanford University School of Medicine, 300 Pasteur Drive, Stanford, CA 94305, USA
* Corresponding author.
E-mail address: ying.jura@gmail.com

Urol Clin N Am 41 (2014) 419–427
http://dx.doi.org/10.1016/j.ucl.2014.04.002
0094-0143/14/$ – see front matter © 2014 Elsevier Inc. All rights reserved.

EVALUATION OF POSTPROSTATECTOMY INCONTINENCE

Evaluation of patients with PPI should begin with a detailed history of lower urinary tract symptoms. The pathophysiology of PPI is variable, and history alone is not sufficient to distinguish between bladder causes (poor compliance, detrusor over-activity, and detrusor underactivity) and outlet causes (sphincteric insufficiency or bladder outlet obstruction with overflow) of incontinence. A bladder diary is useful for quantifying urinary fre-quency, number and severity of incontinence episodes, and functional bladder capacity. It is important to demonstrate leakage on physical examination to confirm the diagnosis of SUI. Leakage should occur during cough or bearing down and cease at the end of the straining maneu-ver. This sign confirms the presence of ISD but is not a definitive test of bladder storage or of voiding function.

INDICATIONS FOR URODYNAMICS

Urodynamics is indicated in the evaluation of PPI if there is a question whose answer can have an impact on treatment algorithm or outcome.

Important questions include the following:

- What is the pathophysiology of the inconti-nence? Is it the result of ISD, detrusor overac-tivity, diminished compliance, and/or bladder outlet obstruction with overflow?
- Is there adequate bladder contractility (to overcome the resistance of a male sling)?
- Is there high-pressure storage due to impaired bladder compliance?
- Is there detrusor overactivity?
- Is there bladder outlet obstruction?
- Is there bladder neck or urethral mobility?

URODYNAMIC FINDINGS AND THEIR RELEVANCE

Multichannel urodynamic studies in men with persistent incontinence after radical prostatec-tomy have shown that ISD is by far the most com-mon finding. ISD is found in approximately 90% of men with PPI. Among men with ISD, however, only 25% to 50% have ISD alone without concomitant bladder dysfunction on urodynamics.[6-8] Detrusor overactivity is found in approximately 30% to 40%, decreased contractility in 30% to 40%, bladder outlet obstruction in 20% to 25%, and decreased compliance in 5% of men undergoing urodynamics for PPI.[7-11] Approximately 15% of patients with PPI demonstrate only bladder dysfunction without ISD.[6-8]

Bladder dysfunction may result from pre-existing outlet obstruction or age-related detrusor overac-tivity or may occur de novo after prostatectomy as a result of bladder denervation or obstruction due to anastomotic stricture. Impaired detrusor contractility, which occurs in 29% to 61% of pa-tients after radical prostatectomy (de novo in approximately 47%), and poor compliance, which occurs in 8% to 39% of patients (de novo in approximately 50%), have traditionally been thought to resolve within 8 months.[12,13]

Treatment options differ depending on the etiology of PPI. The management of postprosta-tectomy SUI is primarily surgical, with options including injection of periurethral bulking agents, male sling, and AUS. Detrusor overactivity should be treated initially with behavioral modification, pelvic floor exercises, and pharmacotherapy (anti-muscarinics or β_3-agonists). In refractory cases, chemodenervation with botulinum toxin injection or neuromodulation may be efficacious. Detrusor underactivity and/or bladder outlet obstruction causing overflow incontinence may require inter-mittent self-catheterization. Diminished bladder compliance can be difficult to treat, usually starting with antimuscarinics and scheduled voiding to prevent high intravesical pressures.

Detrusor Underactivity

Detrusor contractility plays a vital role during micturition, especially after the placement of a potentially obstructing sling. It is an important finding in men with PPI because a weak bladder is a relative contraindication to male sling surgery. Because the male sling is designed to prevent leakage during straining, it follows logically that patients with weak detrusors who rely on abdom-inal straining to facilitate efficient bladder emptying are at higher risk for retention after sling surgery.

The International Continence Society defines detrusor underactivity as a contraction of reduced strength and/or duration, resulting in prolonged bladder emptying and/or a failure to achieve com-plete bladder emptying within a normal period. Detrusor contractility is assessed during the pressure-flow portion of urodynamics but the spe-cific method of evaluation has not been standard-ized, and there are no agreed-on normal values of detrusor pressure during voiding in men who are status postprostatectomy. In most urodynamics studies of patients with PPI, detrusor underactivity has been defined using surrogate measures such as (1) the presence of Valsalva voiding, (2) low detrusor pressure at maximum flow (PdetQmax), or, most commonly, (3) bladder contractility nomograms developed for men with BPH, derived using both urinary flow rates (Qmax) and PdetQmax.[11]

The use of surrogate measures of detrusor contractility based on BPH nomograms, however, can be inaccurate in men after prostate extirpation because of the low outflow resistance state in these men. In such patients, the contractile pressure required to maintain axial flow can approach zero. Thus, PdetQmax can be low due to reduced urethral resistance in patients with ISD and may, therefore, be an inaccurate measure of detrusor strength.

In the setting of PPI due to ISD, a more appropriate measure of detrusor strength is independent of flow and unrelated to urethral resistance and characterizing contractility as a single parameter. Contractility can be represented by a power factor—as a product of detrusor pressure and shortening velocity by the methods described by Griffiths[14] or van Mastrigt.[15] These calculations, however, require complex, computer-assisted analysis of pressure-flow studies. A simpler method of measuring detrusor power is to directly measure bladder muscle contraction pressure under isovolumetric conditions—and, therefore, independent of urinary flow. The best measure of detrusor contraction strength, therefore, is the isometric detrusor contraction pressure (Piso).

One reliable method for obtaining Piso measurement is the mechanical stop test.[10] During voiding, an examiner gently occludes the penile urethra, thereby inhibiting urinary flow but not aborting the bladder contraction. The maximum detrusor pressure reached during this maneuver is the Piso (**Fig. 1**). This mechanical stop test is reproducible and does not inhibit detrusor contraction.[16,17] Piso measurements less than 50 cm H_2O are considered diagnostic of detrusor underactivity.[18,19]

The mechanical occlusion of the outlet is preferred to a volitional interruption of flow; as such, voluntary cessation may underestimate the maximum isometric pressure due to reflex detrusor inhibition induced by the activation of voluntary striated sphincter activity. In addition, it may be difficult or impossible for a patient with detrusor overactivity to stop the urinary stream once it is initiated, especially after prostatectomy with concomitant weakness of the external sphincter mechanism.

Elliott and Comiter[11] retrospectively reviewed the urodynamics findings of 62 men evaluated for PPI and found that 40% had a Piso less than

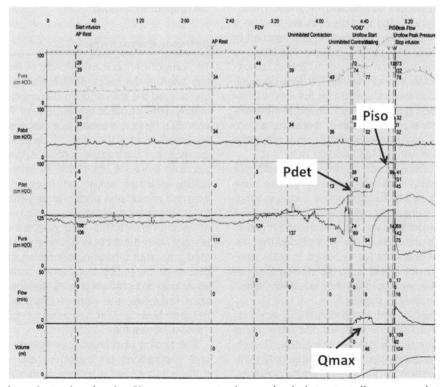

Fig. 1. Urodynamics tracing showing Piso measurement using mechanical stop test: (*heavy arrows*) start of stop test when examiner occludes urethra, thereby stopping flow. Maximal isometric pressure (Piso) is 99 cm water.

50 cm H_2O. They also found that the use of common surrogates for bladder contractility, such as the Bladder Contractility Index (BCI = Pdet Qmax + 5 Qmax) less than 100, which has been validated in men with BPH but not in men devoid of a prostate, and the mere presence of Valsalva voiding were imprecise markers of detrusor underactivity in this population. Rather, the direct measure of bladder contractility independent of urethral sphincteric resistance was necessary to accurately measure true bladder contractility.

Detrusor underactivity is a potentially important finding in men with PPI, because it may be a relative contraindication to certain types of male sling surgery. Because the compressive male sling provides fixed resistance and is designed to prevent leakage with straining, it seems logical that it would interfere with voiding dependent on or augmented by Valsalva. The placement of a potentially obstructive male sling in a patient with detrusor underactivity, therefore, theoretically increases the risk for retention. There are few clinical studies, however, on the effects of the male sling in patients with impaired detrusor contractility or those who void by Valsalva. Han and colleagues[10] performed retrospective review comparing 50 patients after sling placement (AdVance, InVance, and Virtue) with a mean BCI of 70 (range 33–97) with normal controls and found no differences in postvoid residual (PVR), patient satisfaction, or Qmax. The investigators concluded that their results may be a reflection of how bladder function is measured in this population. The authors believe that BCI and its derivatives, however, may not be accurate measures of bladder strength in men with PPI, because Elliott and Comiter[11] showed that the isovolumetric contraction pressure (Piso), which is independent of urethral resistance and, therefore, a pure measure of detrusor contractility, did not differ between men with low and normal BCI.

Detrusor underactivity, however, should not adversely affect surgical success of AUS because the cuff is cycled to an open phase during voiding, with relief of urethral occlusion. In a prospective trial of 40 patient followed for a mean of 53 months, Trigo Rocha and colleagues[20] concluded that the presence of preoperative impaired bladder contractility did not affect surgical outcome. Even pure Valsalva voiding does not adversely affect the outcome of AUS surgery.[21]

In the setting of detrusor underactivity, when an artificial sphincter is not desired, the retroluminal transobturator sling is a viable alternative. The retroluminal transobturator sling provides only minimal compression of the bulbar urethra. Rather, its mechanism of action relies on proximal urethral relocation. The sling is placed retrourethrally, under the proximal urethral bulb, and, on tensioning, facilitates a 2.5- to 3-cm proximal relocation of the bulbar urethra. It is hypothesized that laxity of posterior support predisposes to misalignment of the proximal urethra, contributing to inefficacious coaptation of the urethral sphincter complex.[22] This abnormal anatomy and proximal urethral prolapse that may occur after prostate extirpation may be remedied by a retroluminal sling that can realign the mobile urethral sphincter complex and restored the preprostatectomy configuration. Once the sling is appropriately tensioned, the urethral bulb is proximally relocated into the higher-pressure pelvic outlet by a distance of 2 to 3 cm, which can function as a backstop during straining.[23] In a large cohort of patients with at least 1-year follow-up, Rehder and colleagues[24] demonstrated no change in Pdet, PVR, or flow rate after surgery, supporting this nonobstructive mechanism of action.

More prospective studies using appropriate measures of detrusor contractility independent of urethral resistance are needed to define the risk of urinary retention, obstructive voiding dysfunction, and outcomes of the male sling and AUS in men with postprostatectomy SUI and detrusor underactivity. In the meantime, the AUS and the retroluminal sling are the preferred options for these patients based on the mechanism of action of the respective devices.

Detrusor Overactivity

The rate of detrusor overactivity in men with PPI has been in the range of 30% to 40%.[7,8,25] It is considered the sole or main diagnosis in approximately 10% of patients.[7] In 25% of PPI patients with ISD, there is a secondary diagnosis of detrusor overactivity. The rate of de novo detrusor overactivity postradical prostatectomy is only approximately 5%, with 33% of patients already having detrusor activity at baseline.[25] In men who had presumably normal storage function prior to radical prostatectomy, the urodynamic finding of detrusor overactivity or diminished compliance is most likely due to poor accommodation associated with supraphysiologic infusion of a bladder that has experienced a prolonged underfilled state secondary to continual urinary leakage. With long-term follow-up, the rate of detrusor activity is reduced from 38% at 8 months to approximately 18% at 36 months.

The finding of detrusor overactivity has important implications for treatment and counseling. If the sole or main diagnosis is detrusor overactivity then antimuscarinic medications and other treatments for overactive bladder (β_3-agonist, botulinum toxin, posterior tibial nerve stimulation, and sacral neuromodulation) are the recommended treatment options. If detrusor overactivity is found along with ISD, then it should be taken into consideration during patient counseling but is not an absolute contraindication to AUS or sling placement.

Although the bone-anchored sling and older slings designs work by compressing the urethra, the retrourethral transobturator sling is designed to be nonocclusive. It does not seem to increase voiding pressure or increase the rate of urgency in patients with preoperative findings of detrusor overactivity.[24,26] Studies on the retrourethral transbturator sling, however, have relatively short follow-up (1–3 years).

Preoperative detrusor overactivity does typically improve after AUS implantation and does not adversely affect resolution of SUI. Afraa and colleagues[27] retrospectively reviewed the charts of 16 patients and found that the rate of detrusor overactivity decreased from 50% to 25% after AUS implantation. As discussed previously, men with high-volume SUI have bladders that are chronically underfilled because SUI prevents the accumulation of urine in the bladder. In the most severe cases, these patients may only passively leak and never volitionally void. As a result, medium and even slow-fill cystometry may demonstrate poor accommodation or compliance as well as detrusor overactivity. These findings typically resolve over time after successful SUI surgery and bladder retraining. Despite the likelihood of improvement, persistent overactive bladder symptoms remain common, and patients must be counseled accordingly.[28]

Impaired Compliance

The International Continence Society defines bladder compliance as the relationship between change in bladder volume and change in detrusor pressure.[29] It can be calculated by dividing the change in volume by the change in detrusor pressure during the same time period ($C = \Delta V/\Delta Pdet$). The recommended points for this calculation are the start of infusion to the end of filling and at cystometric capacity. Compliance greater than 20 mL/cm is generally accepted as normal.

De novo reduced bladder compliance has been detected in up to 32% of men after prostatectomy, with persistence in 28% after 36 months.[25] A study examining urodynamic findings with PPI, however, found only a 5% rate of decreased compliance.[8] The presence of impaired bladder compliance is a contraindication to male sling placement due to concerns that the increased voiding pressures

may lead to upper tract compromise. The AUS has been reported to have a predictably high success even in the setting of diminished bladder compliance.[28] Bladder compliance may even improve. In a comparison of pre- and post-AUS implantation urodynamic parameters, Afraa and colleagues[27] revealed statistically significant improvement in bladder capacity from 271 ± 117 to 295.6 ± 151 mL ($P = .05$) and bladder compliance from 7.6 ± 3.95 to 12.5 ± 10.3 mL/cm H_2O ($P = .03$). Voiding pressures are not increased after implantation of the AUS because voiding occurs with the device in the open setting.

In radiated patients, however, it is not safe to assume that impaired compliance necessarily resolves after resumption of normal bladder filling and evacuation cycles. Rather, there may be a component of intrinsic bladder wall fibrosis secondary to radiation-induced obliterative endarteritis.[30] It is important, therefore, to continue to monitor upper tract anatomy to assess for the development of hydronephrosis, which has been reported after AUS placement, and to repeat urodynamics as necessary to assess filling and storage pressures.[31]

Low Abdominal Leak Point Pressure

Although pad use, bother from leakage, and patient preference typically dictate the implementation of surgical treatment, the degree of sphincteric incompetence can also affect the type of treatment recommended for the management of the stress incontinence. The value of abdominal leak point pressure (ALPP) in management of PPI is debatable. There is evidence that patients with higher ALPP, and, therefore, more preserved sphincteric function tend to respond better to periurethral bulking agents than do patients with a lower ALPP. Sanchez-Ortiz and colleagues[32] found that an ALPP less than 60 cm predicts a higher failure rate with periurethral bulking agents compared with those with higher leak point pressures. Twiss and colleagues,[33] however, found no correlation between ALPP and pad weight.

Bladder Outlet Obstruction

Bladder outlet obstruction after radical prostatectomy is most commonly due to persistent bladder neck contracture or urethral stricture. These occur at a rate of 2.7% to 20%.[34,35] Clinically significant anastomotic and urethral strictures are typically diagnosed on cystoscopy. Findings of bladder outlet obstruction on urodynamics should be interpreted with caution. Scarring and relative poor compliance that can develop in a urethra that has been operated on can result in the finding of catheter-induced bladder outlet obstruction. This should be suspected if there is a large difference between the Qmax obtained with and without the 7F urodynamics catheter in place. If an adequate free flow and low PVR can be confirmed, this finding of obstruction on urodynamics is not a contraindication to anti-incontinence surgery.

ROLE OF FLUOROSCOPY (VIDEOURODYNAMICS)

The use of simultaneous fluoroscopy at the time of multichannel urodynamic studies can be useful for determining the degree of proximal urethral and bladder neck mobility. Assessing these parameters is important because the mechanism of action of the retroluminal sling is thought to rely more on repositioning the prolapsed sphincteric urethra than on direct compression of the bulbar urethra. In instances of restricted mobility, a compressive sling or artificial sphincter may be more appropriate.

The repositioning test has been advocated as a predictor of adequate residual sphincter function and predictor of retroluminal sling success.[36] Rehder and colleagues[22] demonstrated that the ALPP increases on gently pushing the preanal midperineum in a cephalad direction (avoiding direct compression of the urethral bulb). On perineal elevation, men with sufficient residual sphincter function (ie, mild ISD) demonstrate passive sphincter closure with cystoscopically visible contraction of the striated sphincter-positive repositioning test.[37] A positive repositioning test preoperatively is predictive of a successful outcome with a retroluminal transobturator sling.[22,36,38]

As an alternative to the repositioning test, fluoroscopic assessment during straining can demonstrate the degree of bladder neck and proximal urethral mobility. Comiter and colleagues[39] reported on a cohort of men with PPI who underwent videourodynamic evaluation. Those men with PPI after surgery alone had significantly more proximal urethral descent with straining than men with PPI who had adjuvant radiation and those with urinary incontinence after radiotherapy alone. Only those men with adequate mobility were offered retroluminal sling surgery, whereas those with more pure ISD were treated with a compressive sling or AUS.

WHEN MAY URODYNAMICS NOT BE NEEDED?

There are some clinical scenarios when urodynamic studies may not be needed for PPI. One situation is if AUS has already been selected as the treatment of PPI based on patient or surgeon preference. AUS offers the best chance of "cure" and the most predictable outcomes. It has a 90% satisfaction rate regardless of the degree of incontinence. Furthermore, bladder dysfunction, like detrusor overactivity, detrusor underactivity, and poor bladder compliance, has been shown to have no impact on the outcome of AUS and may even improve after implantation.[27,28]

In certain clinical situations, there is consensus that AUS represents the best treatment option for PPI. In such instances, urodynamics may not provide any information that would alter treatment recommendation or counseling. There is no question whose answer would alter treatment plan or prognosis. One exception to this recommendation is radiated patients, who may benefit from preoperative urodynamics despite AUS being the treatment of choice.

AUS is best treatment option for high-volume SUI (>450 g leakage/d) where patients with such severe incontinence preoperatively are at higher risk for postoperative incontinence after sling surgery.[40–42] In a prospectively evaluated cohort of 62 patients with PPI treated by a bone-anchored sling, Fischer and colleagues[42] found that leakage of greater than 450 g per day was associated with a substantially lower success rate—from greater than 70% in those with more mild leakage to less than 50% in those with greater than 450 g per day. The AUS is the treatment of choice for most men with high-volume SUI because its success rates are generally independent of the degree of leakage.[43,44] The 1-year results of the initial clinical trial of the Virtue quadratic sling demonstrated that the degree of improvement in leakage with the quadratic sling, which combines proximal urethral relocation (similar to the retrourethral transobturator sling) and perineal urethral compression (similar to bone-anchored slings) may not be adversely affected by the degree of urinary incontinence. Its efficacy does not seem to significantly differ among patients with mild (<100 g/d), moderate (100–400 g/d), or severe (>400 g/d) SUI.[45] More experience with this promising device, however, is necessary to fully evaluate its efficacy in men with high-volume SUI.

AUS is also the treatment of choice for patients who have had previous implantation of an AUS or male sling. Tuvgan and colleagues[46] demonstrated that cure/improved rate of the male sling was inferior to the AUS (25% vs 75%) in a cohort of men with recurrent PPI after previous AUS erosion. Because adequate tissue compliance is necessary for successful urethral compression and/or proximal repositioning with a sling, it is not surprising that radiation, previous AUS explantation, and prior male sling—all of which may result in poorly compliant and relatively noncompressible fibrotic urethra—are associated with diminished efficacy for the noncircumferential male slings.

In men who have failed prior male sling surgery, placement of the AUS remains a straightforward procedure. With prior retrourethral transobturator sling or bone-anchored sling, a surgeon may elect to place the AUS cuff transcrotally, and the previous sling neither renders the operation more difficult nor decreases AUS efficacy.[1,47] The proximal sling device left in situ may then act as a pseudo–double cuff, and the potential morbidity of removing the sling unnecessarily is avoided. With the quadratic sling, which spans the bulbar urethra and perineal urethra, the sling must be excised prior to AUS placement. This, too, can be done in a straightforward fashion, because the sling is readily identified, dissected from the bulbospongiosus, leaving a relatively unscarred urethra that can easily accommodate the AUS cuff.[48]

AUS is also the treatment of choice for patients with a history of radiation, but preoperative urodynamics remains useful in this population. A history of radiotherapy has been shown a risk factor for sling failure in multiple series because of the increased rates of bladder dysfunction.[24,40,49] In a prospective series with 24 radiated patients followed for a median of 18 months after placement of a retrourethral transobturator sling, Bauer and colleagues[50] found only a 25% cure rate and a 25% improvement rate. This is compared with a success rate of almost 80% in patients without a history of prior AUS or sling surgery.[51] Although preoperative urodyanmics may not be needed for deciding among surgical treatment options, it can still be useful for detecting bladder dysfunction to allow early intervention and for counseling in this high-risk population.

SUMMARY

Urodynamics is indicated for the evaluation of PPI unless AUS placement has been predetermined, such as by patient/surgeon preference, severe incontinence, prior radiation, or previous male sling or AUS placement. It is important that urodynamics are only performed when there is a question that can be answered and that answer would affect treatment choice or outcome. Urodynamic findings of detrusor underactivity, overactivity, and reduced compliance are important considerations in deciding how best to treat patients with PPI. In the setting of detrusor hypocontractility, a nonobstructive device is indicated, with the retrourethral transobturator sling recommended for

more mild incontinence and the AUS for more severe incontinence. The finding of detrusor overactivity or diminished compliance (in nonradiated patients) typically resolves after successful SUI surgery with either the AUS or sling as the normal cycle of adequate filling and emptying is reestablished. In radiated patient where diminished compliance may be a result of radiation-induced detrusor fibrosis, storage pressures must be monitored with repeat urodynamic evaluation, and it is essential to periodically study upper tract anatomy to determine the presence or absence of hydronephrosis. Although the severity of incontinence is more appropriately gauged as a function of pad weight rather than leak point pressure, ALPP may be a useful measure of sphincteric competence when considering injection of periurethral bulking agents. Finally, the use of simultaneous fluoroscopy (videourodynamics) can help assess for bladder neck and urethral mobility during straining or during the urethral repositioning test, which is necessary for the preoperative evaluation prior to sling surgery, in order to help decide between a retrourethral and a more compressive sling.

REFERENCES

1. Staskin DR, Comiter CV. Surgical treatment of male sphincteric urinary incontinence. The male perineal sling and artificial urinary sphincter. In: Campbell MF, Kavoussi LR, Novick AC, et al, editors. Campbell-Walsh urology. Philadelphia: WB Saunders; 2006. p. 2391–404.
2. Stanford JL, Feng Z, Hamilton AS, et al. Urinary and sexual function after radical prostatectomy for clinically localized prostate cancer: the Prostate Cancer Outcomes Study. JAMA 2000;283:354–60.
3. Litwin MS, Pasta DJ, Yu J, et al. Urinary function and bother after radical prostatectomy or radiation for prostate cancer: a longitudinal, multivariate quality of life analysis from the Cancer of the Prostate Strategic Urologic Research Endeavor. J Urol 2000;164:1973–7.
4. Nam RK, Herschorn S, Loblaw DA, et al. Population based study of long-term rates of surgery for urinary incontinence after radical prostatectomy for prostate cancer. J Urol 2012;188:502–6.
5. McConnell JD, Barry MJ, Bruskewitz RC. Benign prostatic hyperplasia: diagnosis and treatment. Agency for Health Care Policy and Research. Clin Pract Guidel Quick Ref Guide Clin 1994;(8):1–17.
6. Foote J, Yun S, Leach GE. Postprostatectomy incontinence. Pathophysiology, evaluation, and management. Urol Clin North Am 1991;18:229–41.
7. Groutz A, Blaivas JG, Chaikin DC, et al. The pathophysiology of post-radical prostatectomy

incontinence: a clinical and video urodynamic study. J Urol 2000;163:1767–70.

8. Ficazzola MA, Nitti VW. The etiology of post-radical prostatectomy incontinence and correlation of symptoms with urodynamic findings. J Urol 1998; 160:1317–20.

9. Chung DE, Dillon B, Kurta J, et al. Detrusor underactivity is prevalent after radical prostatectomy: a urodynamic study including risk factors. Can Urol Assoc J 2013;7(1):E33–7.

10. Han JS, Brucker BM, Demirtas A, et al. Treatment of post-prostatectomy incontinence with male slings in patients with impaired detrusor contractility on urodynamics and/or who perform Valsalva voiding. J Urol 2011;186:1370–5.

11. Elliott CS, Comiter CV. Maximum isometric detrusor pressure to measure bladder strength in men with postprostatectomy incontinence. Urology 2012; 80:1111–5.

12. Giannantoni A, Mearini E, Di Stasi SM, et al. Assessment of bladder and urethral sphincter function before and after radical retropubic prostatectomy. J Urol 2004;171:1563–6.

13. Porena M, Mearini E, Mearini L, et al. Voiding dysfunction after radical retropubic prostatectomy: more than external urethral sphincter deficiency. Eur Urol 2007;52:38–45.

14. Griffiths DJ. Assessment of detrusor contraction strength or contractility. Neurourol Urodyn 1991; 10:1–18.

15. van Mastrigt R. Estimation of the maximum contraction velocity of the urinary bladder from pressure and flow throughout micturition. Urol Res 1990;18:149–54.

16. Sullivan MP, DuBeau CE, Resnick NM, et al. Continuous occlusion test to determine detrusor contractile performance. J Urol 1995;154:1834–40.

17. McIntosh SL, Griffiths CJ, Drinnan MJ, et al. Noninvasive measurement of bladder pressure. Does mechanical interruption of the urinary stream inhibit detrusor contraction? J Urol 2003;169:1003–6.

18. Comiter CV, Sullivan MP, Schacterle RS, et al. Prediction of prostatic obstruction with a combination of isometric detrusor contraction pressure and maximum urinary flow rate. Urology 1996;48: 723–9 [discussion: 729–30].

19. Sullivan MP, Yalla SV. Detrusor contractility and compliance characteristics in adult male patients with obstructive and nonobstructive voiding dysfunction. J Urol 1996;155:1995–2000.

20. Trigo Rocha F, Gomes CM, Mitre AI, et al. A prospective study evaluating the efficacy of the artificial sphincter AMS 800 for the treatment of postradical prostatectomy urinary incontinence and the correlation between preoperative urodynamic and surgical outcomes. Urology 2008;71: 85–9.

21. Lai HH, Hsu EI, Teh BS, et al. 13 years of experience with artificial urinary sphincter implantation at Baylor College of Medicine. J Urol 2007;177: 1021–5.

22. Rehder P, Freiin von Gleissenthall G, Pichler R, et al. The treatment of postprostatectomy incontinence with the retroluminal transobturator repositioning sling (Advance): lessons learnt from accumulative experience. Arch Esp Urol 2009;62:860–70.

23. De Ridder D, Rehder P. The AdVance® Male Sling: anatomic features in relation to mode of action. Eur Urol 2011;10:383.

24. Rehder P, Mitterberger MJ, Pichler R, et al. The 1 year outcome of the transobturator retroluminal repositioning sling in the treatment of male stress urinary incontinence. BJU Int 2010;106:1668–72.

25. Giannantoni A, Mearini E, Zucchi A, et al. Bladder and urethral sphincter function after radical retropubic prostatectomy: a prospective long-term study. Eur Urol 2008;54:657–64.

26. Collado Serra A, Resel Folkersma L, Domínguez-Escrig JL, et al. AdVance/AdVance XP Transobturator Male Slings: preoperative degree of incontinence as predictor of surgical outcome. Urology 2013;81: 1034–9.

27. Afraa TA, Campeau L, Mahfouz W, et al. Urodynamic parameters evolution after artificial urinary sphincter implantation for post-radical prostatectomy incontinence with concomitant bladder dysfunction. Can J Urol 2011;18:5695–8.

28. Lai HH, Hsu EI, Boone TB. Urodynamic testing in evaluation of postradical prostatectomy incontinence before artificial urinary sphincter implantation. Urology 2009;73:1264–9.

29. Abrams P, Cardozo L, Fall M, et al. The standardisation of terminology of lower urinary tract function: report from the Standardisation Sub-committee of the International Continence Society. Neurourol Urodyn 2002;21:167–78.

30. Sung DJ, Sung CK. Urinary bladder. In: Kim SH, editor. Radiology illustrated: uroradiology. Berlin, Heidelberg: Springer-Verlag; 2012. p. 721–86.

31. Ghoniem GM, Lapeyrolerie J, Sood OP, et al. Tulane experience with management of urinary incontinence after placement of an artificial urinary sphincter. World J Urol 1994;12:333–6.

32. Sanchez-Ortiz RF, Broderick GA, Chaikin DC, et al. Collagen injection therapy for post-radical retropubic prostatectomy incontinence: role of Valsalva leak point pressure. J Urol 1997;158:2132–6.

33. Twiss C, Fleischmann N, Nitti VW. Correlation of abdominal leak point pressure with objective incontinence severity in men with post-radical prostatectomy stress incontinence. Neurourol Urodyn 2005;24:207–10.

34. Kao TC, Cruess DF, Garner D, et al. Multicenter patient self-reporting questionnaire on impotence,

incontinence and stricture after radical prostatectomy. J Urol 2000;163:858–64.

35. Kundu SD, Roehl KA, Eggener SE, et al. Potency, continence and complications in 3,477 consecutive radical retropubic prostatectomies. J Urol 2004; 172:2227–31.

36. Bauer RM, Gozzi C, Roosen A, et al. Impact of the 'repositioning test' on postoperative outcome of retroluminar transobturator male sling implantation. Urol Int 2013;90:334–8.

37. Bauer RM, Mayer ME, Gratzke C, et al. Prospective evaluation of the functional sling suspension for male postprostatectomy stress urinary incontinence: results after 1 year. Eur Urol 2009;56: 928–33.

38. Rehder P, Berger T, Kiss G, et al. AdVance™ Male Sling: anatomic evidecne of retrourethral position after tensioning without direct urethral compression. European Urology Supplements 2008;7:87.

39. Comiter CV, Payne CK, Vecchiotti R. A prospective analysis of video-urodynamic data to measure urethral mobility in men with post-prostatectomy incontinence. J Urol 2011;185:184–5.

40. Cornu JN, Sebe P, Ciofu C, et al. The AdVance transobturator male sling for postprostatectomy incontinence: clinical results of a prospective evaluation after a minimum follow-up of 6 months. Eur Urol 2009;56:923–7.

41. Rehder P, Haab F, Cornu J, et al. Treatment of postprostatectomy male urinary incontinence with the transobturator retroluminal repositioning sling suspension: 3-year follow-up. Eur Urol 2012;62: 140–5.

42. Fischer MC, Huckabay C, Nitti VW. The male perineal sling: assessment and prediction of outcome. J Urol 2007;177:1414–8.

43. Imamoglu MA, Tuygun C, Bakirtas H, et al. The comparison of artificial urinary sphincter implantation and endourethral macroplastique injection for the treatment of postprostatectomy incontinence. Eur Urol 2005;47:209–13.

44. Silva LA, Andriolo RB, Atallah AN, et al. Surgery for stress urinary incontinence due to presumed sphincter deficiency after prostate surgery. Cochrane Database Syst Rev 2011;(4):CD008306.

45. Comiter CV, Nitti V, Elliot C, et al. A new quadratic sling for male stress incontinence: retrograde leak point pressure as a measure of urethral resistance. J Urol 2012;187:563–8.

46. Tuygun C, Imamoglu A, Gucuk A, et al. Comparison of outcomes for adjustable bulbourethral male sling and artificial urinary sphincter after previous artificial urinary sphincter erosion. Urology 2009;73:1363–7.

47. Comiter CV. The male perineal sling: intermediate-term results. Neurourol Urodyn 2005;24:648–53.

48. Jura YH, Comiter CV. The male sling for postprostatectomy incontinence: current concepts and controversies. In: Graham SD, Keane TE, editors. Glenn's Urologic Surgery. Philadelphia: Lippincott Williams & Wilkins, in press.

49. Cornel EB, Elzevier HW, Putter H. Can advance transobturator sling suspension cure male urinary postoperative stress incontinence? J Urol 2010; 183:1459–63.

50. Bauer RM, Soljanik I, Füllhase C, et al. Results of the AdVance transobturator male sling after radical prostatectomy and adjuvant radiotherapy. Urology 2011;77(2):474–9.

51. Osman NI. Slings in the management of male stress urinary incontinence. Curr Opin Urol 2013; 23:528–35.

Urodynamics in the Evaluation of Female LUTS

When Are They Helpful and How Do We Use Them?

Harriette Scarpero, MD

KEYWORDS

- Lower urinary tract symptoms • Urodynamics • Overactive bladder • Detrusor overactivity
- Voiding dysfunction

KEY POINTS

- Lower urinary tract symptoms do not always correlate with urodynamic diagnoses.
- In mixed urinary incontinence, urodynamics changes the diagnosis more often than in stress or urgency urinary incontinence.
- Storage and voiding lower urinary tract symptoms often coexist.
- Voiding abnormalities on pressure-flow studies can be responsible for significant storage symptoms.
- There are no urodynamic standards for obstruction in women.

INTRODUCTION

Much of the published work about urodynamics provides the best practice guidelines and standards of technique.[1,2] How to appropriately apply urodynamics (when and for what purpose) remains guided mostly by expert opinion. Recent randomized controlled trials seek to guide its use in a well-defined population: women with complaints of stress urinary incontinence (SUI) who demonstrate SUI on physical examination. These important studies should be familiar to all clinicians who perform urodynamics or treat SUI. Despite a greater understanding of when urodynamic testing may be safely omitted in the evaluation of SUI, there remain many clinical scenarios in the treatment of women presenting with lower urinary tract symptoms (LUTS) in which the decision to use urodynamic testing still relies on the clinician's judgment.

Arguments for urodynamics describe it as the best method to diagnose the underlying pathophysiology underlying LUTS. The objective data often direct therapy and help reduce unnecessary surgery or reduce the time and cost spent on unindicated treatments. Arguments against urodynamics are that the test is invasive, costly, and associated with some morbidity. A quality study also requires a well-trained clinician. However, urodynamics remains the most reliable method to confirm a presumptive diagnosis of lower urinary tract dysfunction.

In 2012, the American Urological Association (AUA) in conjunction with the Society of Urodynamics and Female Urogenital Reconstruction (SUFU) published guidelines to assist the clinician in the appropriate selection of urodynamic tests after an appropriate clinical assessment of the patient presenting with LUTS.[3] The discussion points

4320 Harding Road, Suite 521, Nashville, TN 37205, USA
E-mail address: hscarpero@comcast.net

Urol Clin N Am 41 (2014) 429–438
http://dx.doi.org/10.1016/j.ucl.2014.04.010
0094-0143/14/$ – see front matter

to the limitations of literature analysis due to the scarcity of level 1 evidence on the topic. Nineteen guideline statements are provided relating to SUI and pelvic organ prolapse, overactive bladder (OAB), urgency urinary incontinence, mixed urinary incontinence (MUI), neurogenic bladder, and LUTS.

Recent randomized controlled trials include Value of Urodynamic Evaluation (VALUE) and Value of Urodynamics Before Stress Urinary Incontinence Surgery (VUSIS2). The results clarify the use of preoperative urodynamics in a well-defined population of women with clinical pure SUI; however, this information is not generalizable to other groups of women with incontinence.[4,5] High-level evidence to guide the use of urodynamics in voiding LUTS or MUI and OAB is limited. Because randomized controlled trials concern specific populations, the findings may be at odds with the priorities of the clinician who is accountable for the outcome and satisfaction of the individual patient. The decision to perform urodynamics is often based on a desire to assess risk for postoperative complications to better counsel patients on an individualized basis. Although the urodynamics information may not mitigate complications, it may help manage expectations and improve patient satisfaction even if complete cure is not achieved. When treating quality of life conditions for which surgical intervention is elective, patient expectations can be high. If conservative therapy alone is planned, urodynamics can be avoided. If surgical intervention is contemplated, urodynamics may offer valuable counseling information.

An objective diagnosis used to counsel before therapy often has value to the patient. Intuitively, the collection of objective data to establish the correct diagnosis is the first step to effective therapy. One study demonstrated that, when given a choice to have a diagnosis confirmed by urodynamics before proceeding with treatment of urinary incontinence, most women will chose to proceed with urodynamics. In this patient preference study, patients with LUTS were offered treatment based on their preference for conservative therapy based on symptoms or treatment preceded by urodynamics.[6] Women without a preference were randomized to the two options. The investigators found that in this group of 309 women (median age 46 years), 49.4% preferred urodynamics, whereas 18.4% chose conservative therapy alone. Urodynamics did not confer any advantage in treatment response over treatment based on symptoms alone but there was a higher rate of follow-up in those who chose urodynamics. This was also true in the randomized groups. The greater rate of follow-up suggests that urodynamics may improve patient compliance with therapy. Corroborating studies are still needed.

INVESTIGATING LUTS IN WOMEN

LUTS are highly prevalent in men and women; rates are affected by age and ethnic or racial group.[7] Women present with a variety of urinary complaints relating to both bladder storage (urinary incontinence, urgency, frequency, and nocturia) and emptying (urinary retention or incomplete emptying, hesitancy, straining, slow stream, intermittency, and terminal dribbling). In some cases, the presenting complaint, such as recurrent urinary tract infection, may not describe LUTS. However, further discussion of bladder symptoms when taking history may hint that a functional disorder could underlie the presenting complaint. The clinician must use the patient's complaint, medical history, findings on physical examination, and urinalysis to develop the clinical diagnosis.

Despite best efforts at obtaining a thorough and accurate history, LUTS do not always correlate with urodynamic diagnoses.[8,9] Digesu and colleagues[10] published a systematic review of 23 clinical trials relating to 6282 women with incontinence. Results showed that urodynamics confirmed the clinical diagnosis of SUI in 75% of the cases. Clinical SUI was reclassified infrequently as MUI in 9% and as detrusor overactivity (DO) in 7% of the cases. As shown in other studies investigating the use of urodynamics in SUI, there were a small (8%) percentage of women with clinical SUI who had normal urodynamics. This review confirmed the opinion that the clinical diagnosis of SUI is usually made correctly without urodynamics.

Greater rates of change were found in women with clinical MUI, of which 46% were reclassified as SUI and 21% as DO. Based on urodynamics, rates of diagnostic change were greatest in women with clinical MUI. A full two-thirds of these women had the diagnosis changed by urodynamics. Most were found to have pure urodynamic SUI. These results point out that urodynamic findings in MUI are varied, as are the patients' complaints. When there is disagreement between the urodynamic findings and the patient's symptoms, urodynamics findings are not necessarily any more valid than the patient's symptoms. Failure to demonstrate DO or SUI on urodynamics does not wholly exclude either as a source of the patient's symptoms.

A physician must expertly listen and observe during the history and physical examination to recognize symptoms, physical findings, and patterns that point to a high likelihood of a functional urinary disorder. Although there is a role for empiric treatment of many LUTS, when there is a very high clinical suspicion for a functional disorder that may be best treated surgically, diagnostic urodynamic testing may be the prudent next step. Urodynamics is also relied on when empiric treatments fail to provide the expected satisfactory results and the clinician wishes to confirm the clinical diagnosis.

URODYNAMIC TESTS USED TO INVESTIGATE LUTS

Uroflow is a noninvasive screening test for patients with LUTS. It may be used when any voiding abnormality is suspected. A normal flow curve is a smooth arc-shaped curve. The kinetics of the detrusor contraction accounts for the uroflow pattern observed.[1,2] Abnormal flow curves may suggest obstruction or a weak detrusor but they cannot diagnose the true pathophysiology. The uroflow may be altered by a low voided volume or if the patient feels inhibited during voiding; therefore, the clinician should repeat the uroflow in these situations.

Filling cystometrography (CMG), the urodynamic investigation of the pressure-volume relationship of the bladder during filling, provides assessment of bladder sensation, the presence of DO, bladder compliance, and bladder capacity.[1,2] Urethral function studies may also be undertaken during filling CMG. In clinical practice, the presence of altered compliance, DO, or other urodynamic abnormalities detected during CMG may alter the treatment decision, particularly when invasive surgery is planned. Women in whom there is a high index of suspicion for these urodynamic findings should have a CMG performed, including those with urinary urgency incontinence (UUI), retention, neurogenic disease (known or occult), pelvic radiation, or radical pelvic surgery.

A pressure-flow study (PFS) examines the relationship of bladder pressure and urine flow rate during the voiding phase.[1,2] A PFS is useful to diagnose bladder outlet obstruction (BOO)or impaired detrusor contractility in a patient complaining of voiding symptoms and urgency incontinence.

An electromyogram (EMG) is a test of perineal muscle function and measurement of the striated sphincteric muscles of the perineum.[1] In normal voiding, relaxation of the pelvic muscles occurs before the detrusor contraction. Therefore, increases in EMG activity during the voiding phase suggest dysfunctional voiding or detrusor sphincter dyssynergia. EMG is a useful adjunct to PFS to help diagnose voiding dysfunction.

Videourodynamics refers to the simultaneous fluoroscopic imaging of the lower urinary tract during multichannel urodynamics for the purpose of obtaining anatomic data. It may be particularly useful to diagnose a pop-off mechanism of vesicoureteral reflux in the patient with low compliance of the bladder or to determine the level of obstruction in BOO. For the diagnosis of primary bladder neck obstruction, confirmation is made exclusively by fluoroscopy.

Although urodynamic tests are described as separate entities, a thorough urodynamic investigation of a patient with LUTS includes both CMG and PFS. Because clinical symptoms do not predict urodynamic findings, it cannot be relied on that a patient with storage symptoms needs only CMG and a patient with voiding symptoms needs only PFS. The importance of attention to the voiding phase in women is highlighted by a study of women with LUTS in which urodynamic results of CMG were compared with results of CMG and PFS.[11] The investigators found that PFS added relevant information in 33% of women. Seventy percent of the women with PFS findings had normal a CMG. An interesting and thought-provoking finding is that five women initially classified as dysfunctional voiders were later reclassified as having detrusor-external sphincter dyssynergia (DESD) after a neurologic evaluation. All five had also shown DO on CMG. The investigators caution that increased sphincter activity during voiding and DO, especially if associated with DO incontinence in a woman younger than 40 years, should prompt consideration of a neurologic referral. This study emphasizes that storage and voiding symptoms are related, and that voiding abnormalities may result in storage abnormalities, such as low compliance, DO, change in sensation, and change in capacity.

URODYNAMIC TESTING IN FEMALE LUTS

Multichannel urodynamics is the gold standard study for the evaluation of complex LUTS and identification of functional urinary abnormalities. Urodynamic testing is not a screening tool for LUTS. It is a diagnostic tool meant to be applied with precision to patients who have already been identified as having LUTS. Specifically, urodynamics is used to answer a particular question or series of questions regarding the patient's symptoms. The validity of the test to answer these questions is predicated on the ability to reproduce the clinical symptoms during the test. The results should confirm a diagnosis when there is clinical doubt or when therapy may be altered by the findings. If conservative therapy alone is planned, urodynamics may be avoided because there is little risk to the patient from conservative, nonsurgical therapies. Urodynamics may be more helpful before surgical intervention.

Like other diagnostic tests, urodynamics is not infallible nor is it therapeutic or capable of generating a therapeutic decision. Its quality is affected by operator expertise at set up, performance, and interpretation. It is also subject to patient factors, such as the ability to relax and perform to the degree that what she experiences at home can be demonstrated during the study. Assuming ideal operator and patient factors, urodynamics can provide the clinician with data that may change the diagnosis and choice of therapy. It is a commonly held belief that the objective data obtained by urodynamics is superior to clinical impressions and are more important, particularly when the previous clinical diagnosis changes. However, it is not clear that all urodynamic findings are relevant, particularly in the case of DO.

Diagnostic testing does not always predict response to therapy and urodynamics is no different. This is often held up as the rationale for more limited use of urodynamics; however, caution should be used when interpreting this as a repudiation of its use. As pointed out by a committee of experts, "UDS [urodynamic] results are often compared to diagnosis based on clinical symptoms but there is no 'gold standard' to compare to; therefore, estimates of sensitivity, specificity, positive and negative predictive value of UDS are misleading."[12] Quality and value, as they relate to urodynamic testing, have not been clearly defined nor is there a consensus of thought. Stakeholders (physicians, patients, and third-party payers) probably would not have identical definitions in any case.

STORAGE LUTS: SUI

The application of urodynamics has changed more in SUI than any other category of female LUTS. Results of randomized controlled trials published by the Urinary Incontinence Treatment Network (UITN) support the recommendation that urodynamics is not necessary in the preoperative evaluation of pure SUI.[4,13–15] When SUI is described clearly by the patient, urine leak is seen with cough or Valsalva on examination (supine or standing) and there is no sign or symptom of urinary retention, SUI is diagnosed without the need for confirmatory urodynamics. Urodynamics in this situation is thought to only increase cost and delay treatment.

Whether the same recommendation can be made for the patient with persistent or recurrent SUI is not known. Although not specifically addressed in these trials, by similar reasoning, the patient who reports persistent SUI after incontinence surgery and demonstrates leakage on examination may not need urodynamics before undergoing a secondary incontinence procedure, particularly if the treating physician is confident in the clinical diagnosis. However, recurrent SUI in which the patient had a previously successful incontinence procedure but later becomes incontinent may warrant urodynamics before deciding on any future invasive therapy.

Measuring urethral competence tests of abdominal leak point pressure (ALPP) and maximal urethral closure pressure (MUCP) fell out of widespread use with the advent of midurethral polypropylene slings and changes in concepts of intrinsic sphincter deficiency (ISD). Contemporary concepts of ISD recognize it as a spectrum rather than absolute. Because not all women with urethral hypermobility leak, those women who do must have some degree of ISD. Data from the Stress Incontinence Surgical Treatment Efficacy Trial (SISTEr) found that ALPP did not predict surgical outcome, but the Trial of Mid Urethral Slings (TOMUS) results found a higher rate of SUI postoperatively at one year. Women with ALPP or MUCP were in the lowest quartile.[13,16] Although clinicians may still use the sign of leakage with cough or Valsalva to confirm SUI on urodynamics, the absolute pressure required to cause the leak rarely plays a role in the choice of surgery nor does it predict response. Even with urethral bulking agents for SUI, outcomes data support its use in women with urethral hypermobility as well as in the ISD patient.[17] Despite changes in the understanding of SUI within clinical practice, documentation of an ALPP less than or equal to 100 cm water is still routinely required in order for the Center for Medicare Services to approve a bulking agent for SUI. Therefore, if a Medicare patient with SUI desires a bulking agent as treatment, she will require urodynamics first.

It is well documented that urodynamics fails to diagnose urodynamic incontinence in a small percentage of women with SUI symptoms. Almost 12% of women in SISTEr and TOMUS had absence of urodynamic SUI (USUI) despite clinical symptoms and a positive standardized empty bladder stress test.[18] In TOMUS, prolapse reduction testing was not performed, which certainly affected the rate of USUI detection.

In a secondary analysis of these studies, high-grade pelvic organ prolapse (stage 3–4) was strongly associated with the absence of USUI. The investigators noted that the urodynamic bladder capacity (maximum cystometric capacity) in these women was lower, which may reflect that they did not reach the volume at which they leak in their own environment.[18] Given the supraphysiologic filling and room-temperature fluid for urodynamics, some women do not accommodate as large a bladder volume as they do naturally, thus they fail to demonstrate leakage. Management of women with clinical SUI but no USUI is problematic. These patients were at higher risk for postoperative urgency urinary incontinence in a secondary analysis of the VALUE trial.[19]

When clinical SUI exists with pelvic organ prolapse, demonstrable with or without prolapse reduction, urodynamics is not needed to confirm or guide the treatment of incontinence. The decision to treat is based on the patient's reported bother from incontinence. More controversial is the use of urodynamics to diagnose occult SUI in women who have no symptoms of SUI. Methods of prolapse reduction are not standardized and results can be affected by the method used. Currently, clinicians must be guided by their own level of comfort in the possibility of de novo SUI versus a potential complication from a sling that may not have been necessary.

STORAGE LUTS: MUI AND OAB

MUI is a very common condition affecting 45% of adults identified as having OAB and incontinence in the NOBLE (National Overactive Bladder Evaluation) study.[20] The cause of MUI is unknown and a common pathophysiologic link may exist between UUI and SUI.[21] Despite it being very prevalent, not all MUI is the same, and definitions vary. MUI can refer to equal stress and urge symptoms, stress predominant symptoms, urge predominant symptoms, USUI with DO, and USUI with clinical urge symptoms but no DO. With all the variety of definitions of MUI, interpreting the data from various studies is difficult. Although MUI includes all of these combinations, there is no well-recognized standard for reporting the condition of MUI. Even among the experienced centers within the UITN, diagnoses of OAB were decreased after urodynamics, presumably due to failure to demonstrate DO.[19] The presence of urgency symptoms along with SUI has long been a confounding factor in the decision to proceed with incontinence surgery. MUI symptoms are regarded as more complex than pure SUI, and DO is often considered a risk for poorer surgical outcome. Women with MUI show greater levels of bother and higher levels of incontinence than those with pure SUI or UUI.[22,23] Given the mixed urodynamic findings and negatives associated with MUI, urodynamics is traditionally advocated in patients with MUI,

particularly when the patient is not aware of which symptom (stress or urge) is predominant.

In a large study that sought to define the urodynamic diagnoses of women with MUI, 49% of 3338 women reported MUI symptoms and were studied urodynamically.[10] Women with stress predominant MUI demonstrated USUI in 82% of urodynamics. Detrusor overactivity was diagnosed in 64% of women with urge predominant symptoms. In women with equal stress and urge symptoms, 46% had DO and 54% had USUI on urodynamics. Nineteen percent showed both USUI and DO.

Although urodynamics in MUI may reveal information that would reduce unnecessary surgery and complications, it may fail to identify DO in up to 40% of women with MUI or OAB symptoms.[22,24] Furthermore, the absence of DO on urodynamics does not exclude it as the cause of symptoms. Traditionally, patients with DO are offered treatments for OAB before proceeding with surgery for SUI. Whether the diagnosis of DO portends a negative impact on SUI surgery is debatable.

Various studies have reported conflicting results regarding the effect of DO on surgical outcome. Several smaller studies have shown urge symptoms resolve in a sizable percent of patients with MUI after pubovaginal sling.[25,26] Nevertheless, when urge symptoms persist or worsen after incontinence surgery, patient satisfaction is greatly reduced. The holy grail of MUI remains identification of the clinical or urodynamic parameter that can consistently predict either resolution or persistence of urgency after surgery. Some investigators have noted that high amplitude DO (>15–25 cm water) portends poorer surgical results with persistent urgency.[27,28] In SISTEr, preoperative and postoperative rates of DO did not predict the likelihood of successful SUI outcome or the risk of postoperative voiding dysfunction.[29] However, preoperative and postoperative urgency incontinence symptoms (MESA [medical epidemiological and social aspects of aging] urge index score) were some of the factors negatively associated with long-term continence rates in extended follow-up of SISTEr.[30]

The AUA-SUFU Guideline Diagnosis and Treatment of OAB (Nonneurogenic) in Adults states as a clinical principle that urodynamics should not be used in the initial workup of the uncomplicated patient.[31] In other words, urodynamics should not be a routine investigation for patients who present with OAB symptoms. In patients with either OAB that fails to respond to conservative measures and pharmacotherapy, urodynamics may confirm the clinical diagnosis and exclude an unrecognized finding such as impaired bladder compliance or a voiding abnormality. In the absence of an unexpected urodynamics finding, DO may or may not be found on urodynamics in patients with OAB. However, its presence is not necessary to define the condition nor to proceed with a variety of treatments. Giarenis and colleagues[22] examined differences in women with OAB according to whether urodynamics demonstrated DO. DO was detected in 43% of women. Baseline characteristics of age, body mass index, and hormonal status were no different between the groups. Women with DO showed a significantly smaller cystometric capacity and lower bladder compliance than the non-DO group. There was no difference in the rates of SUI diagnosed in each group; however, 62 subjects with DO could not be assessed for SUI due to the severity and persistence of their uninhibited detrusor contractions. Quality of life in the groups was assessed and validated, and the presence of DO had a statistically significant negative effect on scores.[22] With such diversity of symptoms and urodynamic findings, MUI and refractory OAB remain entities for which urodynamics remains an important diagnostic tool.

VOIDING LUTS: SUSPECTED OBSTRUCTION

Voiding symptoms are less common in women than storage symptoms but may occur in conjunction with storage symptoms or alone in an important segment of women presenting for urologic care. The prevalence of voiding symptoms in women is informed by a large cross-sectional prevalence study of urinary symptoms in men and women in the United States, United Kingdom, and Sweden. Within the study population, 5.2% of women older than age 40 years had voiding symptoms, and 14.9% reported both storage and voiding symptoms.[32] The EPIC study, a population-based study of bladder symptoms in over 19,000 subjects in Canada and Europe found that two-thirds of women complained of LUTS with 51.3% complaining of storage symptoms and 19.5% complaining of voiding symptoms.[33] In both studies, voiding symptoms presented in conjunction with storage symptoms more often than alone.

Women with voiding complaints may complain of straining to void, having to stand to void, intermittency of voiding, constant suprapubic pressure, or irritative symptoms, including urgency, frequency, and incontinence. Some women with urinary frequency and urgency may report that they are not sure that they completely empty; however, this may be due to their urge recurring shortly after their void or the failure to lose the urge after a void. Therefore, OAB symptoms may give the false sensation of failure to empty. The converse may also occur. Failure to empty may lead to bothersome frequency, urgency, and incontinence.

Many studies evaluating obstruction after incontinence surgery demonstrate that irritative symptoms may be the primary symptom related to obstruction.[34,35] Given the variety of presenting complaints, the evaluating physician must take a careful history and have a high index of suspicion for obstruction when the differential diagnosis warrants.

True emptying abnormalities may occur in women due to obstruction from previous incontinence surgery, other pelvic surgery, high-grade pelvic organ prolapse, or, more rarely, urethral disease, such as stricture, neoplasm, diverticulum, or cyst (**Table 1**). These conditions produce anatomic obstruction. Antecedent pelvic surgery for prolapse or incontinence may be all that is needed to determine that a patient is obstructed, particularly if the clinician has knowledge of preoperative urinary symptoms and voiding parameters. In this situation, the strong temporal relationship of the surgery to the onset of voiding symptoms is implication of the surgery. Urodynamic studies in this case may or may not show characteristic high-pressure and low-flow voiding. Therefore, it may not change the surgeon's decision to release the sling. Cystoscopy may be helpful in determining if urethral disease is present or, if a urethral abnormality is noted on physical examination, other testing such as voiding cystourethrogram (VCUG) or urethral MRI may be used.

Obstruction may also be due to functional causes such as dysfunctional voiding, detrusor sphincter dyssynergia, or primary bladder neck obstruction. Functional obstruction is not associated with visible anatomic changes in the lower urinary tract and cannot be diagnosed without a functional study such as urodynamics.

URODYNAMIC TESTING IN SUSPECTED OBSTRUCTION

The role of urodynamics in obstruction after incontinence surgery is debatable. The woman who is in persistent retention after a sling without any other cause for her retention can easily be diagnosed with an obstructing sling. Therefore, urodynamics

Table 1
Causes of female voiding LUTS: obstruction

Bladder Outlet Obstruction	
Functional	Dysfunctional voiding or DESD Primary bladder neck obstruction
Anatomic	Urethral disease Previous incontinence surgery High-grade pelvic organ prolapse

before sling lysis in this patient is not necessary. When the patient who is not in frank urinary retention presents with voiding complaints several years after an incontinence surgery, it is difficult for the clinician to know whether the surgery is obstructing or whether those symptoms are related to another cause.

The Urodynamic Guidelines state that clinicians may perform a postvoid residual urine volume (PVR) in patients with LUTS as a safety measure to rule out significant urinary retention both initially and during follow-up (clinical principle).[3] PVR is a simple test that may be useful in women with voiding LUTS. It is a measurement that may be obtained noninvasively with a bladder scan or by simple catheterization when a bladder scanner is unavailable. A PVR of greater than 100 mL is regarded as abnormal but the value reveals nothing about the cause. Another limitation is that voiding symptoms have not been shown to be predictive of an elevated PVR. In a study of 636 women, voiding symptoms had a low sensitivity and specificity for elevated PVR.[36] When using PVR as a screening tool for LUTS, a single reading may be insufficient to deem the PVR abnormal. A second corroborating measurement of PVR is prudent; or more than two to establish a trend in PVR measurements. Some asymptomatic patients may have PVR greater than 100 mL, so this parameter in isolation may be inconsequential. Additionally, a normal PVR should not exclude a patient with bothersome voiding LUTS from further investigation or treatment.

An uninstrumented uroflow is also a useful screening tool in the evaluation of a woman with voiding symptoms and the possibility of obstruction. It is a noninvasive measure that reports flow velocity, flow pattern, and voiding time. Abnormalities from normal values can point to possible voiding dysfunction, yet it is not specific for cause. Whether the cause is due to the bladder outlet or to the detrusor cannot be determined from an uninstrumented uroflow. Its greatest use is as a comparison to the flow achieved on a PFS. If the uninstrumented flow is a normal bell-shaped curve, abnormalities on the PFS must be interpreted with caution. Abnormalities on the PFS can be related to the intraurethral catheter and some studies have demonstrated that increased outlet resistance can reduce the flow rate and lead to overdiagnosis of bladder outlet obstruction.[37,38]

When the clinical question posed is whether or not the woman with voiding LUTS is obstructed, the PFS is the urodynamic test that can answer the question and make a definitive diagnosis. The PFS has the ability to distinguish bladder outlet obstruction (BOO) from impaired detrusor contractility. The filling cystometry phase of full urodynamics may also be relevant. Detrusor overactivity is often associated with obstruction; however, other cystometric findings of compliance and capacity may also help understand the patient's symptoms; particularly because the storage and voiding symptoms often coexist. When the clinician has a high index of suspicion for BOO, urodynamics should be performed.

In other conditions, such as SUI and OAB, urodynamics is not recommended before conservative therapy. In the case of voiding symptoms, obstruction and detrusor underactivity are distinctly different in cause and management. Delay in distinguishing obstruction that could potentially be corrected surgically could lead to unnecessary bother for patients. In the treatment of suspected BOO, conservative treatment may simply be management by clean intermittent catheterization. This can be undertaken without urodynamics; however, it is invasive and unpopular in most neurologically intact patients. Because no satisfactory pharmacotherapy exists and physical therapy is only useful for functional causes, surgery may be the only option for correction. Given the paucity of conservative options for BOO, a convincing argument can be made for urodynamics early in the evaluation of women with suspected BOO.

Performance and interpretation of urodynamics for female voiding symptoms is hampered by a lack of information on normative values for voiding in women and a lack of standardized urodynamic criteria to define obstruction in women. There is more variability in voiding in women than in men. Some women generate a detrusor contraction to void, whereas others may just relax the pelvic floor. Many women void normally with a low detrusor pressure, whereas some augment voiding or void exclusively with abdominal straining. Urodynamic standards for obstruction in men and the nomograms based on these standards cannot be applied to women.

Several studies have sought to establish urodynamic parameters to define obstruction in women. Definitions are usually based on detrusor pressure and flow rate.[39–42] Broad application of these definitions has been limited. Nitti and colleagues[43] defined BOO on videourodynamics by the fluoroscopic images of the bladder outlet during voiding. These investigators rightfully point out that "if normal voiding occurs at a low detrusor pressure, then bladder response to obstruction by the generation of higher voiding pressures may be difficult to perceive."[43] The addition of simultaneous fluoroscopic imaging of the bladder outlet during

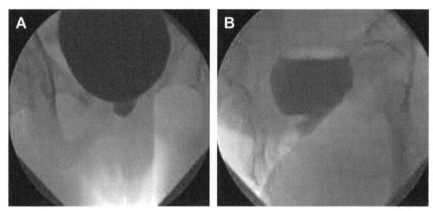

Fig. 1. The fluoroscopic appearance of "spinning top urethra". The image (*A*) is an anterior posterior view and the image (*B*) shows an oblique view. The appearance is similar in cases of dysfunctional voiding and DESD. In both cases the bladder neck and proximal urethra appear dilated to the level of the external sphincter.

voiding aids the diagnosis and helps localize the site of obstruction. Their definition of BOO is radiographic evidence of obstruction between the bladder neck and distal urethra in the presence of a sustained detrusor contraction without application of strict pressure-flow criteria. In the 331 women studied, PFSs were not sufficient to diagnose BOO in all women. Although a helpful adjunct for the diagnosis of BOO, fluoroscopy in the urodynamics suite is not universally available.

Akikwala and colleagues[44] published an interesting study of 154 women with clinical obstruction who underwent urodynamics and compared rates of BOO based on five different definitions: three PFS cutoff criteria, videoourodynamic criteria, and the Blaivas-Groutz nomogram.[42] The greatest concordance was found between the fluoroscopic criterion and pressure-flow cutpoints; whereas the Blaivas-Groutz nomogram overestimated obstruction compared with other criteria. There are no absolute urodynamics values that can be used to reliably diagnose BOO in women, so the evaluation must be individualized. Urodynamic findings consistent with obstruction are supported when a combination of history, physical, PVR, and uroflow are also highly suggestive of a voiding abnormality.

FUNCTIONAL URINARY OBSTRUCTION

BOO related to functional causes, such as dysfunctional voiding, primary bladder neck obstruction (PBNO), and DESD, may also be diagnosed by urodynamics. Both dysfunctional voiding and DESD describe involuntary contraction of the external urinary sphincter during voiding, but DESD occurs in a patient with a suprasacral spinal cord lesion. Dysfunctional voiding is demonstrated on EMG by increased activity on the voiding

phase. Unfortunately, EMG is easily influenced by artifact, which can affect interpretation. It is important for the clinician to correlate the EMG findings to the patient's symptoms. Increased EMG activity during voiding in a patient without voiding complaints may be due to discomfort voiding with the catheter in place or inhibition related to voiding in an artificial setting and in front of the examiner. Performance of additional fill and emptying phases may help corroborate findings or help clarify what is artifact. On a practical note, simply asking the patient whether the void was similar to her voids at home is also helpful to determine whether the increased EMG activity is authentic or artifact.

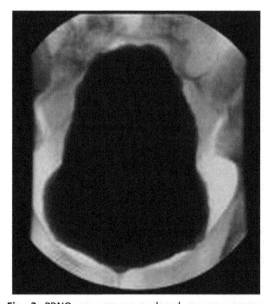

Fig. 2. PBNO appears as a closed or very narrow bladder neck. It is often described as a bird-beak bladder for this reason.

The fluoroscopic appearance of dysfunctional voiding is similar to DESD. In both cases, the bladder neck and proximal urethra appear dilated to the level of the external sphincter. This fluoroscopic appearance is referred to as a spinning top (**Fig. 1**). In contrast, PBNO appears as a closed or very narrow bladder neck. It is often described as a bird-beak bladder for this reason (**Fig. 2**). Urodynamics without concomitant fluoroscopy cannot definitively diagnose the level of obstruction. Although not ideal, when videourodynamics is not available, cystoscopy can be used to rule out an anatomic obstruction and a VCUG can be obtained if the cystoscopy is negative.

SUMMARY

Urodynamics should be used selectively in women with LUTS to answer specific functional questions. Diagnostic and management dilemmas are often encountered in the treatment of women with LUTS. The use of urodynamics has been clarified in one specific population, that of women with pure SUI symptoms. In that population, it is safe to forego urodynamics preoperatively. In many other groups of women with bothersome LUTS, urodynamics remains the best test available to confirm a diagnosis and exclude others. New guidelines in urodynamics and nonneurogenic OAB state that empiric treatment should not be withheld for urodynamics first for the patient with uncomplicated OAB. Urodynamics is more aptly reserved for the OAB patient who fails to respond to empiric conservative therapy or in whom there is a concern for a poorly compliant bladder or urinary obstruction. In the case of voiding LUTS, the current literature points to the value of voiding studies to better understand both the filling and emptying function.

REFERENCES

1. Schafer W, Abrams P, Liao L, et al. Good urodynamic practices: uroflowmetry, filling cystometry, and pressure-flow studies. Neurourol Urodyn 2002; 21:261–74.
2. Abrams P, Cardozo L, Fall M, et al. The standardisation of terminology in lower urinary tract function: report from the standardisation sub-committee of the International Continence Society. Urology 2003; 61:37–49.
3. Winters JC, Dmochowski RR, Goldman HB, et al. Adult urodynamics: AUA/SUFU guideline. J Urol 2012;188(Suppl 6):2464–72.
4. Nager CW, Brubaker L, Litman HJ, et al. A randomized trial of urodynamic testing before stress-incontinence surgery. N Engl J Med 2012; 366:1987–97.
5. Leijsen SA, Kluivers KB, Mol BW, et al. Value of urodynamics before stress urinary incontinence surgery. Obstet Gynecol 2013;121(5):999–1008.
6. Majumdar A, Latthe P, Toozs-Hobson P. Urodynamics prior to treatment as an intervention: a pilot study. Neurourol Urodyn 2010;9:522–6.
7. Coyne KS, Sexton CC, Bell JA, et al. The prevalence of lower urinary tract symptoms (LUTS) and overactive bladder (OAB) by racial/ethnic group and age: results from OAB-POLL. Neurourol Urodyn 2013; 32:230–7.
8. Kuo HC. Clinical symptoms are not reliable in the diagnosis of lower urinary tract dysfunction in women. J Formos Med Assoc 2012;111:386–91.
9. Leijsen SA, Hoogstad-van E, Mol BWJ, et al. The correlation between clinical and urodynamic diagnosis in classifying the type of urinary incontinence in women. A systematic review of the literature. Neurourol Urodyn 2011;30:495–502.
10. Digesu GA, Salvatore S, Fernando R, et al. Mixed urinary symptoms: what are the urodynamic findings? Neurourol Urodyn 2008;27:372–5.
11. Carlson KV, Fiske J, Nitti VW. Value of routine evaluation of the voiding phase when performing urodynamic testing in women with lower urinary tract symptoms. J Urol 2000;164:1614–8.
12. Bosch JL, Cardozo L, Hashim H, et al. Constructing trials to show whether urodynamic studies are necessary in lower urinary tract dysfunction. Neurourol Urodyn 2011;30:735–40.
13. Nager CW, Fitzgerald MP, Kraus SR, et al. Urodynamic measures do not predict stress continence outcomes after surgery for stress urinary incontinence in selected women. J Urol 2008;179(4): 1470–4.
14. Kirby AC, Nager CW, Litman HJ, et al. Preoperative voiding detrusor pressures do not predict SUI surgery outcomes. Int Urogynecol J 2011;22(6): 657–63.
15. Lemack GE, Kraus S, Litman H, et al. Normal preoperative urodynamic testing does not predict voiding dysfunction after Burch colposuspension versus pubovaginal sling. J Urol 2008;180:2076.
16. Nagar CW, Sirls L, Litman HJ, et al. Baseline urodynamic predictors of treatment failure one year after mid urethral sling surgery. J Urol 2011;186(2):597–603.
17. Herschorn S, Steele DJ, Radomski SB. Follow up of intraurethral collagen for female stress urinary incontinence. J Urol 1996;156(4):1305–9.
18. Lemack GE, Litman HJ, Nager C, et al. Preoperative clinical, demographic, and urodynamic measures associated with failure to demonstrate urodynamic stress incontinence in women enrolled in two randomized clinical trials of surgery for stress urinary incontinence. Int Urogynecol J 2013;24:269–74.

19. Sirls LT, Richter HE, Litman HJ, et al. The effect of urodynamic testing on clinical diagnosis, treatment plan and outcomes in women undergoing stress urinary incontinence surgery. J Urol 2013;189:204–9.

20. Stewart WF, Van Rooyen JB, Cundiff GW, et al. Prevalence and burden of overactive bladder in the United States. World J Urol 2003;20:327–36.

21. Lai HH, Simon M, Boone TB. The impact of detrusor overactivity on the management of stress urinary incontinence in women. Curr Urol Rep 2006;7:354–62.

22. Giarenis I, Mastoroudes H, Srikrishna S, et al. Is there a difference between women with or without detrusor overactivity complaining of symptoms of overactive bladder? BJU Int 2013;112:501–7.

23. Chou EC, Blaivas JG, Chou LW, et al. Urodynamic characteristics of mixed urinary incontinence and idiopathic urge urinary incontinence. Neurourol Urodyn 2008;27:376–8.

24. McGuire EJ, Cespedes RD. Urodynamic evaluation of stress incontinence. Urol Clin North Am 1995;22:551–5.

25. Serels SR, Rackley RR, Appell RA. Surgical treatment for stress urinary incontinence associated with Valsalva induced detrusor instability. J Urol 2000;163:884–7.

26. McGuire EJ, Lytton B. Pubovaginal sling procedure for stress incontinence. J Urol 1978;119:82–4.

27. Lockhart JL, Vorstman B, Politano VA. Anti-incontinence surgery in females with detrusor instability. Neurourol Urodyn 1984;3:201–6.

28. Schrepferman CG, Griebling TL, Nygaard IE, et al. Resolution of urge symptoms following sling cystourethropexy. J Urol 2000;164:1628–31.

29. Kraus S, Lemack G, Sirls L, et al. Urodynamic changes associated with successful stress urinary incontinence surgery: is a little tension a good thing? Urology 2011;78:1257–62.

30. Richter H, Brubaker L, Stoddard A, et al. Patient related factors associated with long-term urinary continence after Burch colposuspension and pubovaginal fascial sling surgeries. J Urol 2012;188(2):485–9.

31. Gormley EA, Lightner DJ, Burgio KL, et al. Diagnosis and treatment of overactive bladder (non-neurogenic) in adults: AUA/SUFU guideline. J Urol 2012;188(Suppl 6):2455–63.

32. Monz B, Chartier-Kastler E, Hampel C, et al. Patient characteristics associated with quality of life in European women seeking treatment for urinary incontinence: results from PURE. Eur Urol 2007;51:1073–82.

33. Irwin DE, Milsom I, Hunskaar S, et al. Population-based survey of urinary incontinence, overactive bladder, and other lower urinary tract symptoms in five countries: results of the EPIC study. Eur Urol 2006;50(6):1306–14.

34. Starkman JS, Scarpero H, Dmochowski RR. Methods and results of urethrolysis. Curr Urol Rep 2006;7(5):384–94.

35. Starkman JS, Duffy JW, Wolter CE, et al. The evolution of obstruction induced overactive bladder symptoms following urethrolysis for female bladder outlet obstruction. J Urol 2008;179(3):1018–23.

36. Lowenstein L, Anderson C, Kenton K, et al. Obstructive voiding symptoms are not predictive of elevated postvoid residual urine volumes. Int Urogynecol J Pelvic Floor Dysfunct 2008;19(6):801–4.

37. Turker P, Kilic G, Tarcan T. The presence of transurethral cystometry catheter and type of stress test affect the measurement of abdominal leak point pressure (ALPP) in women with stress urinary incontinence (SUI). Neurourol Urodyn 2010;29:536–9.

38. Groutz A, Blaivas JG, Sassone AM. Detrusor pressure uroflowmetry studies in women: effect of a 7Fr transurethral catheter. J Urol 2000;164(1):109–14.

39. Chassagne S, Bernier PA, Haab F, et al. Proposed cutoff values to define bladder outlet obstruction in women. Urology 1998;51(3):408–11.

40. Lemack GE, Zimmern PE. Pressure flow analysis may aid in identifying women with outflow obstruction. J Urol 2000;163(6):1823–8.

41. Defreitas GA, Zimmern PE, Lemack GE, et al. Refining diagnosis of anatomic female bladder outlet obstruction: comparison of pressure-flow study parameters in clinically obstructed women with those of normal controls. Urology 2004;64(4):675–9.

42. Blaivas JG, Groutz A. Bladder outlet obstruction nomogram for women with lower urinary tract symptomatology. Neurourol Urodyn 2000;19(5):553–64.

43. Nitti V, Tu LM, Gitlin J. Diagnosing bladder outlet obstruction in women. J Urol 1999;161(5):1535–40.

44. Akikwala TV, Fleischman N, Nitti VW. Comparison of diagnostic criteria for female bladder outlet obstruction. J Urol 2006;176(5):2093–7.

Urodynamics in the Evaluation of the Patient with Multiple Sclerosis
When Are They Helpful and How Do We Use Them?

Benjamin E. Dillon, MD[a], Gary E. Lemack, MD[b],*

KEYWORDS

• Multiple sclerosis • Urinary tract dysfunction • Urodynamic studies

KEY POINTS

• Lower urinary tract dysfunction and urinary symptoms are common in patients with multiple sclerosis (MS), and when studied, most symptomatic patients will have abnormal urodynamic findings.
• Urologic symptoms may not always predict urodynamic study findings.
• Invasive pressure-flow urodynamic studies may be helpful in providing an accurate diagnosis; however, the universal recommendation of obtaining invasive urodynamic testing in MS patients with minimal to moderate urologic symptom burden seems flawed.

INTRODUCTION

Multiple sclerosis (MS) is an autoimmune inflammatory disease that results in damage to the myelin sheaths of the nerves in the central nervous system. MS is commonly diagnosed between the ages of 20 and 40 and affects women 3 times more often than men. Reportedly, 80% to 96% of all patients with MS will seek urologic care because of bothersome lower urinary tract symptoms (LUTS) at some point in their disease course, and as many as 12% may have symptoms before their actual diagnosis.[1,2] For the purposes of this review, all patients are considered who have LUTS secondary to MS as having neurogenic lower urinary tract dysfunction (NLUTD). Another term that is commonly used in this population is neurogenic bladder (NGB). In the strictest of senses, patients with NGB suffer from some type of bladder dysfunction secondary to an underlying neurologic condition, although this terminology is commonly applied to a broader range of dysfunctions.

Urinary urgency, frequency, and urgency incontinence are the most common symptoms reported by patients with MS, occurring in 37% to 99% of patients.[3] Voiding symptoms (hesitancy, feeling of incomplete emptying, and occasionally urinary retention) are also common in this population, occurring in 34% to 79% of patients.[3,4] Traditionally, filling cystometry combined with pressure/flow studies (that will be now referred to as urodynamic studies or UDS) have been a cornerstone of the initial evaluation of patients with NLUTD, although recently that practice has been challenged. In this review article, the role of UDS in the diagnosis and management of patients with MS is focused on, along with data published within the past 15 years.

a Department of Urology, Kelsey-Seybold Clinic, 2727 West Holcomb, Houston, TX 77005, USA; b Department of Urology, University of Texas Southwestern Medical Center, 5323 Harry Hines Boulevard, Dallas, TX 75390-9110, USA
* Corresponding author.
E-mail address: Gary.Lemack@utsouthwestern.edu

Urol Clin N Am 41 (2014) 439–444
http://dx.doi.org/10.1016/j.ucl.2014.04.004
0094-0143/14/$ – see front matter © 2014 Elsevier Inc. All rights reserved.

URODYNAMIC FINDINGS IN PATIENTS WITH MS

Among patients with MS, the most common UDS finding is neurogenic detrusor overactivity (NDO)[3] seen in up to 70% of patients, although considerable variation exists depending on the population studied. It is theorized that in patients with MS, NDO results from the loss of inhibitory cortical influence of brain stem activity. In contrast, the cause of idiopathic detrusor overactivity (IDO), which represents detrusor overactivity (DO) seen in patients without known neurologic conditions, is less clear, although myogenic, undiagnosed neurogenic, and ischemic causes have all been suggested. Data from a recent study suggest that, in-line with the above physiologic explanation, DO seen in MS differs from that seen in nonneurogenic patients. In 2006, Lemack and colleagues[5] investigated the differences between NDO in MS patients and IDO in patients without any neurogenic cause. The authors examined amplitude of first involuntary detrusor contraction (IDC), maximal detrusor contraction, and threshold volume for the first IDC as a measure severity of DO. Patients with MS and NDO had significantly higher amplitude of first IDC (28.3 cmH$_2$O vs 20.5 cmH$_2$O, P = .003). Similarly, NDO patients had a significantly higher maximal detrusor contraction, 46.4 cmH$_2$O, as compared with IDO patients, 30.8 cmH$_2$O (P = .002). Last, the threshold volume for DO was greater in the MS patients (186.8 mL vs 150.5 mL, P = .037), which the authors attributed to the larger postvoid residual (PVR) in the MS patients. These findings were in concert with a 1997 study by Gray and colleagues,[6] who also noted that patients with MS had higher amplitudes of IDCs as compared with nonneurogenic controls. In addition, MS patients had higher PVRs when compared with nonneurogenic patients.

Others have similarly found DO to be the most common urodynamic finding followed by detrusor sphincter dyssynergia (DSD) (25%), although the variance in prevalence rates between this and other studies reflects the importance of recognizing the particular population surveyed, and the urodynamic definitions used.[7] A recent meta-analysis of the evaluation and management of LUTS in MS noted NDO (25%–100%) and DSD (3%–71%) as the most common UDS findings. Detrusor underactivity or acontractility was seen in 8% to 70%, and altered compliance was found in 7% to 10% of patients.[8]

URINARY SYMPTOMS IN PATIENTS WITH MS

As NDO is the most common UDS finding seen in patients with MS, numerous studies have shown that storage symptoms (such as urgency, frequency, and urgency incontinence) are the most common LUTS reported by these patients. Depending on the population surveyed and the survey tool used, a prevalence of 10% to 100% for LUTS has been reported. Hennessey and colleagues[9] investigated urinary, fecal, and sexual dysfunction in patients with MS. Of 191 patients queried, 53% reported bothersome urologic symptoms, with symptoms of urinary frequency and urgency being much more prevalent than voiding/emptying symptoms. Specifically, some degree of urinary frequency was observed in 177 of 191 (93%) patients. Overall, 145 of 191 (76%) were noted to void more than 5 times a day and 32 of 191 (17%) more than 10 times a day. Interestingly, in this group, 71% of patients reported some degree of urgency incontinence. Chronic catheter use was fairly infrequent in this group. Although 55 of 221 (25%) patients had required the use of a urinary catheter at some point in their disease process, only 6 of 221 (3%) used clean intermittent catheterization on a regular basis.[9] A recent study of 66 patients noted storage symptoms to be more common than emptying symptoms. Specifically, urinary urgency was the most common symptom (65%), followed by frequency (44%) and urgency incontinence (42%).[7]

Although both LUTS and UDS findings are subject to change over time, the LUTS progression does not seem to be inevitable in patients with MS. A 2001 study retrospectively evaluated 22 patients with MS and LUTS over a 14-year period.[10] All patients underwent 2 or more UDS during this time as a means of studying their LUTS. Fourteen of the 22 (64%) patients had stable or worsening of the same symptoms at follow-up and 8 of 22 (36%) had new symptoms of incontinence, obstructive, or irritative symptoms. Six of the 14 patients who did not develop new urinary symptoms were found to have significant changes in UDS patterns, including altered compliance. The data from this small study are not sufficient to conclude that repeated urodynamic investigations are warranted in patients without change in symptoms, baseline renal or urodynamic abnormalities, or patients deemed to be at high risk.

In summary, UDS may be helpful in identifying the type of NLUTD in patients with MS. NDO is the most common UDS observation in symptomatic patients, and storage symptoms, such as urinary urgency and frequency, are the most common symptoms described. Still, the relationship between urinary symptoms and UDS findings in patients with MS requires further scrutiny.

THE COMPLEX RELATIONSHIP BETWEEN DISEASE SEVERITY, UROLOGIC SYMPTOMS, AND URODYNAMIC FINDINGS

The relationship between LUTS, neurologic symptom severity, and UDS findings has been reported on several occasions. Overall, the results are decidedly mixed. Several studies have shown a positive correlation between Expanded Disability Status Scale (EDSS) and NLUTD. A 1999 study retrospectively investigated 116 patients with MS and NLUTD.[11] All patients had EDSS scoring (mean EDSS was 6.0 ± 2.2) and were evaluated with a UDS. UDS abnormalities were noted in 104 of 116 (90%) patients. DO was seen in 94 of 104 (81%) and detrusor acontractility in 4 of 104 (3%). Altered compliance was observed in 12 (10%) patients, whereas detrusor external sphincter dyssynergia was noted in 49 (42%) patients. There was a significant relationship between urologic complaints and neurologic complaints. Specifically, there was a significant positive correlation between the presence of DO and EDSS score ($P = .003$).

In 2001, Barbalias and colleagues[12] prospectively investigated 110 patients with MS with the aim of correlating the response to treatment, the prevailing UDS findings, and severity of disease. All patients had videourodynamics (VUDS; UDS with simultaneous fluoroscopic imaging) and assessment of their MS symptoms using the Kurtzke score, which grades severity of MS symptoms on a scale of 1 (self-sufficient with minimal impact on daily life) to 3 (wheelchair-dependent or nonambulatory). The authors found no correlation between VUDS finding (DSD, DO, altered compliance) and severity of MS.

Onal and colleagues[13] reported on the relationship between urologic symptoms (not UDS findings) and neurologic parameters in patients with MS. The authors retrospectively examined 249 patients with MS and LUTS. Disease severity was determined by EDSS score, whereas urologic symptoms were evaluated using the Boyarsky symptom index, and a questionnaire graded 0 to 22. The authors found only a weak correlation between EDSS scores and storage, voiding and total symptom scores. Because this seldom-used questionnaire lacks specific questions regarding urgency incontinence and the need to strain with urination, the lack of correlation may not be entirely unexpected.

Most recently, Wiedemann and colleagues[14] sought to define which demographic factors were critical in the determination if UDS were necessary in patients with MS. The authors examined 100 patients with MS (9 primary progressive

multiple sclerosis, 47 relapse remitting multiple sclerosis [RRMS], and 43 secondary progressive multiple sclerosis), whose mean EDSS was 4.52 ± 2.26. Sixty-one patients reported urinary incontinence based on recall, with 78.7% of patients reporting that they used incontinence pads. During UDS, 26 patients were observed to have DSD, of which all patients had concomitant DO. Isolated DO was noted in 21 patients. When regression analysis was performed, the highest probability to detect pathologic findings on UDS was seen in patients with an EDSS greater than 6.5 (wheelchair-dependent), followed by use of more than one incontinence pad and having any form of MS other than RRMS. The authors concluded that all patients with MS should be questioned about LUTS and have a UDS if they have increasing degree of disability (EDSS>6.5), use more than one pad per day, or have primary or secondary progressive forms of MS.

Haverkorn and colleagues[15] examined the role of the Urinary Distress Inventory Short Form (UDI-6), a validated questionnaire assessing LUTS, to predict UDS findings of women with MS. They retrospectively reviewed their MS database for patients who had both UDS data and UDI-6 data (n = 68). The authors concluded that aggregate UDI-6 score did not correlate with UDS findings. However, question 1 of the UDI-6 ("Do you experience, and, if so, how much are you bothered by frequent urination?") correlated with filling phase abnormalities, whereas question 5 ("Do you experience, and, if so, how much are you bothered by difficulty emptying your bladder?") correlated with an abnormal PVR.[16] In addition, patients with moderate/severe bother associated with frequency (Q1) were more likely to have DO than those with no/mild bother ($P = .05$), had significantly lower voided volumes (195 mL vs 317 mL, $P = .008$), and lower maximum bladder capacity (293 mL vs 481 mL, $P = .026$). Patients with greater bother while voiding (Q5) were not more likely to have DSD, but did have higher PVR volumes (146 mL vs 52 mL, $P = .036$). Abnormal scoring on these 2 items may indicate that underlying UDS abnormalities are likely to be present.

Dillon and colleagues[17] reported on the ability of UDS to predict the progression of LUTS in patients with MS. The authors retrospectively examined their neurogenic database and identified 122 women who had undergone UDS and had 2 sets of UDI-6 questionnaires, separated by at least 6 months. UDS parameters that were investigated were presence of DO, presence of DSD, maximum cystometric capacity, maximum flow (Qmax), PVR, and presence of urodynamic-proven urge urinary incontinence. The authors found that not only was there a lack of symptom progression in patients who did not have DO or DSD, but after the institution of care at a urologic tertiary referral center, patients had improvement in their symptoms. Patients who were noted to have DO or DSD did not appear, on average, to have an inevitable progression of symptoms.

Although several studies have shown a positive relationship between some clinicodemographic factor of MS and UDS findings or LUTS, others have failed to show a correlation between neurologic symptoms and UDS findings. Nakipoglu and colleagues[7] investigated the correlation between MS symptoms and UDS findings. One hundred thirty-two patients with MS were evaluated over a 1-year period, of which 52 were included in the final analysis. MS symptoms were assessed using EDSS score. UDS abnormalities were seen in 58% of patients, whereas 42% of patients with MS had normal UDS. No relationship was found between disease characteristics and urinary symptoms, urinary complications, and UDS findings ($P>.05$).

Urinary symptoms may also not be predictive of UDS findings, particularly in patients with voiding disorders. In a UDS investigation of patients with neurogenic outlet obstruction due to MS, Lemack and colleagues[18] found that many patients with a UDS finding of a voiding disorder were referred with largely storage type urinary symptoms. Overall, 127 women with MS were evaluated and 108 had UDS. Most patients (52%) were referred for LUTS (urgency, frequency, and/or urgency incontinence). The remainder of the patients was referred for symptoms of voiding dysfunction (21%), suspected UTI (13%), or other complaints (14%). The authors found that there were no differences in chief complaints of those with and without bladder outlet obstruction (BOO), suggesting that if the finding of BOO would impact management, then UDS studies may be necessary to establish the diagnosis, because obstructive symptoms were present less frequently than storage symptoms.

Because of the lack of a clear relationship between symptoms and urodynamic findings, as well as the lack of agreement as to the clinical meaningfulness of demonstrating certain urodynamic findings (ie, it is not clear that demonstrating DO impacts management of patients with OAB symptoms), it remains up to the clinician to decide when UDS are indicated. It is the opinion of the authors that patients with elevated PVR (>150 mL), patients that have failed at least 2 trials of medical therapy, patients with primarily obstructive symptoms (straining, hesitancy), and patients with any degree of hydronephrosis do merit an initial UDS. Furthermore, although the authors do think that patients with MS contemplating stress urinary incontinence surgery should undergo UDS preoperatively, those considering onabotulinumtoxinA injections may not require anything beyond symptom and PVR assessment in most circumstances.

URODYNAMICS AND UPPER TRACT MONITORING

Available studies investigating the prevalence of upper urinary tract (UUT) abnormalities in patients with MS are limited. Furthermore, the relevant clinical question, that is, who, in particular seems to be at greatest risk, has been studied infrequently. Dogma suggests that UDS is essential in the initial evaluation of all patients with MS and LUTS to assess risk factors for UUT damage and implement strategies to prevent damage. This review solely highlights those studies investigating upper tract deterioration and the potential relationship with MS characteristics.

The extent to which the kidneys are at risk for deterioration, as they seem to be for spinal cord injury, has been debated. In a study of 92 patients with MS, the mean creatinine clearance was found to be normal at 132.8.[19] When stratified based on type of MS (relapsing vs progressive), severity of MS based on EDSS score and UDS findings, no significance was found between groups and the rate of upper tract damage based on creatinine clearance. A trend was noted in patients who had severe MS (EDSS>5) and those who had upper tract damage, as defined by a change in serum creatinine levels. Others have demonstrated that patients with MS are at low risk for upper tract deterioration. In a recent series, only 16.7% of MS patients demonstrated some degree of abnormality on renal ultrasound, with focal caliectasis being most common.[20] Findings on UDS were not associated with abnormal ultrasound findings. In a subsequent study by the same authors, patients with concomitant NDO and bladder outlet dyssynergia were not found to have an appreciable difference in detrusor pressures when compared with patients with NDO alone.[18] This finding again gives merit to the fact that even in patients with bladder outlet dysfunction, the incidence of upper tract damage is low. Similarly, Onal and colleagues[13] reported that 5% of their patients with MS were found to have unilateral or bilateral hydronephrosis. Furthermore, no correlation was found between UDS diagnosis and UUT deterioration ($P>.05$).

More recently, Fletcher and colleagues[21] investigated the prevalence of renal ultrasound abnormalities over time in MS patients with LUTS. The authors defined UUT damage as the presence of hydronephrosis, caliectasis, cortical scarring, or stone formation. Over a 9-year period, 173 patients had both UDS and renal ultrasound. Eighty-nine patients had repeat UDS at a time point greater than 12 months. Of these, 5.8% of subjects had abnormalities at initial ultrasound, whereas at follow-up, renal ultrasound (RUS) abnormalities were seen in 12.4% of patients. Overall, there were 7 patients who developed new abnormalities. Of those who developed UUT abnormalities, patients who were greater than 49 years old were more likely to have RUS abnormalities ($P = .04$) as were patients who had abnormal compliance ($P = .04$) on initial UDS evaluation. The authors concluded that the development of UUT abnormalities as determined by RUS overall is low, although older patients and those with abnormal compliance may merit closer supervision.

SUMMARY

NLUTD and urinary symptoms are quite common in patients with MS, and when studied, most symptomatic patients will likely have abnormal UDS findings. This truism does not mean that patients with MS universally require UDS. Therefore, although symptoms may not always predict UDS findings, a combination of noninvasive studies and a stepwise approach to symptomatic management may suffice when treating most patients with LUTS and MS. Thus, for the typical female patient with normal PVR and urgency symptoms, initiating medical therapy seems justified without the need for UDS. There is no doubt that for many, ultimately UDS may be helpful in providing an accurate diagnosis, guiding management decisions, and potentially, offering prognostic information on risk for upper tract deterioration (which is overall quite uncommon). However, the universal recommendation of obtaining UDS in MS patients with minimal to moderate urologic symptom burden seems flawed.

REFERENCES

1. Eikelenboom MJ, Killestein J, Kragt JJ, et al. Gender differences in multiple sclerosis: cytokines and vitamin D. J Neurol Sci 2009;286(1–2):40–2.
2. Radziszewski P, Crayton R, Zaborski J, et al. Multiple sclerosis produces significant changes in urinary bladder innervation which are partially reflected in the lower urinary tract functional status-sensory nerve fibers role in detrusor overactivity. Mult Scler 2009;15(7):860–8.
3. de Seze M, Ruffion A, Denys P, et al. The neurogenic bladder in multiple sclerosis: review of the literature and proposal of management guidelines. Mult Scler 2007;13(7):915–28.
4. Del Popolo G, Panariello G, Del Corso F, et al. Diagnosis and therapy for neurogenic bladder dysfunctions in multiple sclerosis patients. Neurol Sci 2008;29(Suppl 4):S352–5.
5. Lemack GE, Frohman EM, Zimmern PE, et al. Urodynamic distinctions between idiopathic detrusor overactivity and detrusor overactivity secondary to multiple sclerosis. Urology 2006;67(5):960–4.
6. Gray R, Wagg A, Malone-Lee JG. Differences in detrusor contractile function in women with neuropathic and idiopathic detrusor instability. Br J Urol 1997; 80(2):222–6.
7. Nakipoglu GF, Kaya AZ, Orhan G, et al. Urinary dysfunction in multiple sclerosis. J Clin Neurosci 2009;16(10):1321–4.
8. Cetinel B, Tarcan T, Demirkesen O, et al. Management of lower urinary tract dysfunction in multiple sclerosis: a systematic review and Turkish consensus report. Neurourol Urodyn 2013;32: 1047–57.
9. Hennessey A, Robertson NP, Swingler R, et al. Urinary, faecal and sexual dysfunction in patients with multiple sclerosis. J Neurol 1999;246(11):1027–32.
10. Ciancio SJ, Mutchnik SE, Rivera VM, et al. Urodynamic pattern changes in multiple sclerosis. Urology 2001;57(2):239–45.
11. Giannantoni A, Scivoletto G, Di Stasi SM, et al. Lower urinary tract dysfunction and disability status in patients with multiple sclerosis. Arch Phys Med Rehabil 1999;80(4):437–41.
12. Barbalias GA, Liatsikos EN, Passakos C, et al. Vesicourethral dysfunction associated with multiple sclerosis: correlations among response, most prevailing clinical status and grade of the disease. Int Urol Nephrol 2001;32(3):349–52.
13. Onal B, Siva A, Buldu I, et al. Voiding dysfunction due to multiple sclerosis: a large scale retrospective analysis. Int Braz J Urol 2009;35(3):326–33.
14. Wiedemann A, Kaeder M, Greulich W, et al. Which clinical risk factors determine a pathological urodynamic evaluation in patients with multiple sclerosis? An analysis of 100 prospective cases. World J Urol 2013;31(1):229–33.
15. Haverkorn RM, Fletcher SF, Lemack GE. Evaluating women with multiple sclerosis and neurovesical dysfunction: is urodynamic testing always necessary? In The Society of Urodynamics and Female Urology Annual Meeting. Las Vegas, 2009.
16. Uebersax JS, Wyman FF, Shumaker SA, et al. Short forms to assess life quality and symptom distress for urinary incontinence in women: the incontinence impact questionnaire and the urogenital distress inventory. Neurourol Urodyn 1995;14:131–99.

17. Dillon BD, Haverkorn RH, S Murray, et al. Urodynamic predictors of lower urinary tract symptom progression in multiple sclerosis: do specific findings predict those destined to progress, in The Society of Urodynamics and Female Urology Annual Meeting. Phoenix, 2011.

18. Lemack GE, Frohman E, Ramnarayan P. Women with voiding dysfunction secondary to bladder outlet dyssynergia in the setting of multiple sclerosis do not demonstrate significantly elevated intravesical pressures. Urology 2007;69(5):893–7.

19. Krhut J, Hradilek P, Zapletalova O. Analysis of the upper urinary tract function in multiple sclerosis patients. Acta Neurol Scand 2008;118(2):115–9.

20. Lemack GE, Hawker K, Frohman E. Incidence of upper tract abnormalities in patients with neurovesical dysfunction secondary to multiple sclerosis: analysis of risk factors at initial urologic evaluation. Urology 2005;65(5):854–7.

21. Fletcher SG, Dillon BE, Gilchrist AS, et al. Renal deterioration in multiple sclerosis patients with neurovesical dysfunction. Mult Scler 2013;19(9):1169–74.

Neurogenic Lower Urinary Tract Dysfunction
How, When, and with Which Patients Do We Use Urodynamics?

Teresa L. Danforth, MD[a],*, David A. Ginsberg, MD[b]

KEYWORDS

- Neurogenic bladder • Spinal cord injury • Myelodysplasia • Urodynamics • Autonomic dysreflexia

KEY POINTS

- Neurogenic lower urinary tract dysfunction (NLUTD) affects a large population of patients with variable bladder behaviors depending on extent of disease.
- Videourodynamics can be useful to evaluate outlet and upper tracts during filling and voiding.
- Monitoring blood pressure during urodynamics (UDS) for autonomic dysreflexia is especially important for patients with spinal cord injury (SCI).
- UDS in patients with NLUTD are challenging because of the inherent lack of sensation and lack of correlation of symptoms to upper tract disease.
- Patients with SCI undergo a period of spinal shock after injury usually lasting 4 to 6 weeks; initial study should be delayed until after bladder reflexes return.

WHO: EPIDEMIOLOGY OF NEUROGENIC LOWER URINARY TRACT DYSFUNCTION

Neurogenic lower urinary tract dysfunction (NLUTD) (also referred to as neurogenic bladder [NGB]) is a condition in which neurologic disease manifests by alteration of bladder and sphincter activities through abnormal bladder innervation. NLUTD affects a large population of patients suffering from various conditions, including spinal cord injury (SCI), stroke, traumatic brain injury, brain tumor, meningomyelocele, cerebral palsy, multiple sclerosis, disk disease, Parkinson disease, and other diseases with long-term neurologic dysfunction, such as diabetes, pernicious anemia, and tabes dorsalis. Bladder behavior in each subset of patients is unique depending on

extent and length of disease and may require close monitoring for symptomatic control and evaluation for potential upper tract deterioration.

Historical Perspective

Before the late 1970s, it was well recognized that patients with NGB developed bladder dysfunction and obstructive uropathy slowly in the first 5 years after injury, followed by a faster progression to eventual renal failure, hypertension, stone formation, incontinence, vesicoureteral reflux (VUR), autonomic dysreflexia (AD), and even death.[1] The recognition that bladder storage pressure is related to upper tract damage was first published in 1978 by Light and colleagues,[2] who reported upper tract deterioration in children with myelodysplasia. This

Disclosures: None (T.L. Danforth), Allergan consultant (D.A. Ginsberg).
[a] Department of Urology, SUNY Buffalo School of Medicine and Biomedical Sciences, Buffalo General Hospital, 100 High Street, Suite B280, Buffalo, NY 14203, USA; [b] Department of Urology, Keck School of Medicine of USC, University of Southern California, 1441 Eastlake Avenue, Suite 7416, Los Angeles, CA 90089-9178, USA
* Corresponding author.
E-mail address: danforth@buffalo.edu

Urol Clin N Am 41 (2014) 445–452
http://dx.doi.org/10.1016/j.ucl.2014.04.003
0094-0143/14/$ – see front matter © 2014 Elsevier Inc. All rights reserved.

was followed by the more familiar work of McGuire and colleagues,[3] in 1981, who described more definitively that myelodysplastic children with elevated detrusor leak point pressure (DLPP) are at risk to develop upper tract disease. This landmark study evaluated 42 pediatric subjects with spinal dysraphism. These subjects underwent urodynamics (UDS) and 68% of subjects with a DLPP greater than 40 cm of water were found to have VUR and 81% had dilated upper tracts on excretory urography. In contrast, none of the subjects with a DLPP less than 40 cm of water had VUR and only 9% had dilation of upper tracts. Subsequently, in 1989, Ghoniem and colleagues[4] described the relationship between high DLPP and poor bladder compliance leading to renal dysfunction, thus prompting the use of pharmacologic therapy in conjunction with intermittent catheterization or procedures, such as bladder neck incision, to decrease outlet resistance.

HOW: PERFORMING UDS IN A PATIENT WITH NLUTD
Preparation for the Study

Many patients with NLUTD also have neurogenic bowel with a home bowel regimen. If the patent is not on a bowel regimen, bowel evacuation may be necessary before the study to allow for accurate rectal catheter pressure readings.[5] If patients are already on a bowel program, rectal suppositories or enemas should be administered with enough time before the study to allow the medication to take effect and avoid bowel movements during the procedure.

The study can be performed in the supine, sitting, or standing positions, or during ambulation.[6] Many patients with NLUTD have limitations in mobility, not allowing them to sit or stand at a commode. These patients do not usually void into a toilet and, therefore, it is acceptable to do the study in the supine position during the test. Patients should be comfortable regardless of position and care should be taken to avoid excess pressure on the limbs and to protect skin from breakdown. If patients volitionally void, the study should be performed in the position in which they usually void (standing or sitting) to allow for optimal pressure-flow measurement. If using fluoroscopy, it is ideal that the patient is positioned so that oblique images can be captured to adequately visualize the bladder neck. To perform the pressure-flow portion of the study, urine may be collected into a wide-bore drainpipe with length to reach the flowmeter. Multiple positions might be required, especially when expected results are not achieved in the supine position.

Filling Rate

Patients with NLUTD tend to be more sensitive to the speed of filling. A voiding diary is often helpful to determine if the filling rate should be decreased. A voiding diary that reveals low volumes and/or consistent leakage with or between each void or catheterization warrants lower filling rates. Generally, starting at a low rate of 10 mL/min or less is advised.[7] If no increase in detrusor pressure is seen, the rate may be increased slowly. If the detrusor pressure continues to increase with filling, decreasing the filling rate or stopping the infusion can help determine if the increase in pressure is due to a detrusor contraction or impaired compliance. In a child with NLUTD, the rate can be calculated as 2% to 10% of the child's age-related bladder capacity.[8,9] Filling rates greater than 20% of estimated bladder capacity have been shown to artificially raise detrusor pressures.[10]

Electromyography

Electromyography (EMG) during UDS is very useful in patients with NLUTD because it may confirm denervation of the pelvic floor musculature or identify discoordination of the external urethral sphincter. In patients with sensation, pad surface electrodes can be placed around the anus. The surface EMG is described as an indirect measure of external sphincter activity. Needle electrodes that more directly assess sphincter function are often used with patients with SCI who have no sensation.[11]

EMG is especially important in evaluation of patients with neurologic lesions suggestive of detrusor external sphincter dyssynergia (DESD) or other evidence of impaired bladder emptying. DESD is seen during the voiding phase of the UDS (Fig. 1). During DESD, the external (voluntary) sphincter contracts (signified by increased EMG activity on UDS), which impairs the ability to empty the bladder by obstructing the outlet and may prevent a sustained bladder contraction, further impairing bladder emptying. EMG is also useful in monitoring patients who have undergone sphincterotomy (see later discussion).

Videourodynamics

Fluoroscopic imaging at the time of videourodynamics allows for the visual evaluation of the entire urinary tract during filling and voiding phases of the study. This imaging identifies anatomic and functional abnormalities of the urinary tract. Fluoroscopy may be performed on a radiograph table in the supine position, or in an radiograph-compatible UDS chair. Patients with NLUTD often

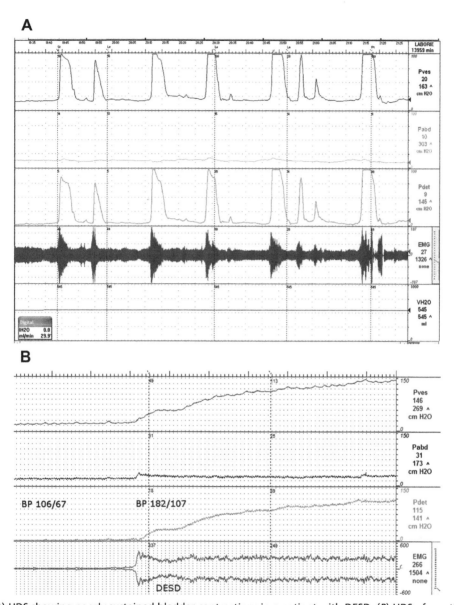

Fig. 1. (A) UDS showing poorly sustained bladder contractions in a patient with DESD. (B) UDS of a patient with AD and DESD. DESD, detrusor external sphincter dyssynergia; EMG, electromyelogram; Pabd, abdominal pressure; Pdet, detrusor pressure; Pves, vesical pressure.

have symptoms that are difficult to differentiate or they may be asymptomatic given their altered sensation. This is particularly challenging in patients with incontinence and incomplete bladder emptying, especially in aging men with benign prostatic enlargement or women with pelvic organ prolapse in whom other causes of dysfunction may be considered.

AD

In 1860, the first case of AD was described by Hilton[12] as hot flushes in a patient with C5 SCI.

Subsequent reports described a variety of symptoms, including hot flushes, sweating with bradycardia, and increase in blood pressure associated with a distended bladder.[13,14] In 1947, Guttman and Whitteridge[15] more fully described the autonomic response after distension of the abdominal viscera leading to effects on cardiovascular activity in subjects with SCI.

AD occurs in approximately 60% of cervical and 20% of thoracic SCI patients. The most common cause is bladder or rectal distension, either spontaneous or by instrumentation (ie, UDS). Other causes include plugged catheters, urinary tract stones, long bone fracture, decubitus ulcers, or even electroejaculation.

A classic sign of AD is an increase in blood pressure with bradycardia, although true bradycardia is seen in only approximately 10% of patients.[16] In fact, tachycardia or no significant change in heart rate is more common in patients with AD. Other signs may include cardiac arrhythmias, changes in skin temperatures (vasodilation above the spinal cord lesion, vasoconstriction below the spinal cord lesion), or changes in mentation.

Common symptoms include sweating above the spinal cord lesion, pounding headache, hot flushes, piloerection, nasal congestion, dyspnea, and anxiety. Although we usually think of patients presenting with these classic symptoms, some patients may be entirely asymptomatic. A study by Linsenmeyer and colleagues[17] demonstrated that 35 of 45 subjects with SCI above T6 were asymptomatic with a significant elevation of blood pressure. This emphasizes the importance of monitoring blood pressure during procedures in patients at risk for AD because significant changes in heart rate and blood pressure may be missed in an asymptomatic patient with possible devastating outcomes, including seizures, stroke, or even death. During UDS, it is generally recommended to obtain a baseline blood pressure and cycle the blood pressure during regular intervals throughout the study (see **Fig. 1**B).

When AD is recognized, the first course of action should be removal of the stimulus. Usually this means ensuring that a patient's catheter is draining correctly, checking for fecal impaction, or (if performing a urologic procedure) stopping and immediately emptying the bladder. It is also recommended to move the patient upright and remove any tight clothing or constrictive devices.[18] If this does not alleviate symptoms and/or decrease blood pressure, the urologist can move to pharmacologic agents.

No particular pharmacologic agent is preferred for acute AD. Multiple drugs have been used, including nifedipine, nitrates, captopril, terazosin, prazosin, phenoxybenzamine, and prostaglandin E2. Nifedipine, a calcium channel blocker, has been the most popular pharmacologic agent for management of acute AD. The usual dose is 10 mg oral and the patient is asked to chew and swallow the medication for optimal absorption. The use of nifedipine is falling out of favor for patients without SCI secondary to adverse events seen in management of hypertensive emergencies, including stroke, heart attack, severe hypotension, and death.[19] Nitrates have been used for acute AD but should be used with caution because of drug interaction, especially in patients who use phosphodiesterase 5 inhibitors. Topical nitrates are easy to use and can be removed quickly if necessary. Typically, they are placed on the shoulders or arms, above the level of injury. If a patient has a history of AD, consideration of prophylaxis given 30 minutes before a urologic procedure, including UDS, would be appropriate (**Fig. 2**).

Patients with recurrent AD can be managed prophylactically. Terazosin, nightly, at 5 mg has been used without change in blood pressure or erectile function.[20] Vaidyanathan and colleagues[21] titrated

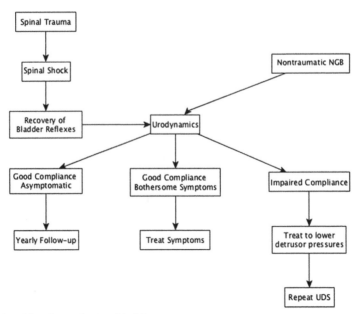

Fig. 2. Treatment algorithm for patients with AD.

terazosin from 1 to 10 mg daily in 18 subjects with resolution of AD in all subjects. One subject required discontinuation secondary to dizziness.

Although prophylaxis has been effective in prevention of AD, it is important to continue to monitor during any urologic procedure, including UDS. Other prophylactic medications include prazosin and phenoxybenzamine. Intravesical botulinum toxin and capsaicin have been demonstrated to decrease AD episodes but further studies are required. If conservative measures do not alleviate AD, sacral denervation has been described; however, studies are conflicting on its effectiveness for eliminating AD. If prophylaxis does not adequately manage AD, the study can be performed under general anesthesia with close monitoring.

Challenges of UDS in NLUTD

UDS in patients with NLUTD may present challenges not seen in neurologically intact patients. For example, many patients with NLUTD lack symptoms because of impaired or altered bladder sensation, or it may be difficult for the patient to define symptoms, such as timing of incontinence. Patients with NLUTD may have a difficult time describing whether leakage is associated with urinary urgency or stress maneuvers, such as transferring in and out of a wheelchair. We know that degree of symptoms does not necessarily correlate with findings on UDS in the neurologically intact patient, which also applies to patients with NLUTD. Importantly, the severity of symptoms does not always correlate with the magnitude of disease affecting the urinary tract.[22–26] This is particularly crucial to remember in patients at risk of upper tract deterioration, such as children with spinal dysraphism. Dator and colleagues[22] demonstrated a poor correlation between neurologic signs and symptoms and UDS assessment in 54 children with myelodysplasia. In addition, although we know that certain levels of injury in patients with SCI tend to have certain types of bladder dysfunction, the exact status of the both the bladder and sphincter behavior cannot be inferred solely from the neurologic evaluation.[23,24] The importance of doing high-quality studies in subjects with NLUTD cannot be overstated because it is the only reliable indicator of the potential risk to upper tract deterioration and the optimal tool to guide appropriate lower urinary tract management.

WHEN: BASELINE AND FOLLOW-UP STUDIES
Spinal Shock

Patients who experience an acute neurologic incident, such as a stroke, traumatic brain injury, or SCI, often develop detrusor areflexia from cerebral shock or spinal shock. Cerebral shock is poorly understood and development of urinary retention in stroke patients is likely multifactorial.[27] These patients are often elderly and carry multiple comorbidities as well as poor mobility, inability to communicate, impaired bladder sensation, and overdistention of the bladder. Return of bladder function is often unpredictable and has not been shown to have correlation with type or severity of stroke.[28]

In 1750, Whytt first described spinal shock as a loss of sensation accompanied by motor paralysis with gradual recovery of reflexes.[29,30] The term shock was first used by Hall and colleagues[31] in 1841 in their work with frogs. Although the mechanism of shock is unclear, the timing of return of reflexes has been well described.[32] The bulbocavernosus reflex and anal wink may never disappear or they may reappear hours after injury, whereas return of reflexive bladder function usually takes at least 4 to 6 weeks. Incomplete spinal cord lesions may recover function in shorter periods of time, such as days or weeks.[33]

Initial Study

Timing of the initial UDS study in patients with an acute neurologic injury depends on the return of their bladder reflexive function. Performing UDS during the spinal shock phase only necessitates another study once bladder function recovers. Recovery of bladder function often manifests with incontinence between catheterizations as well as with new onset of lower extremity spasms.[27] If a patient does not develop incontinence, waiting 3 months after injury is usually adequate with the patient performing intermittent catheterization.

Recommendations for the timing of UDS in children with spinal dysraphism is not well defined. The International Consultation on Incontinence has the only recommendations about UDS in children, stating that "to help identify children at risk for subsequent urinary tract deterioration or a changing neurologic picture, initial UDS studies early in the neonatal period are recommended for children with myelodysplasia or occult spinal dysraphism."[34] They go on to state that all patients with spinal dysraphism should undergo UDS and that timing and technique should be determined on an individual basis.

Follow-up Studies

It is recommended that patients with NLUTD have a yearly follow-up for symptom check. There is no current recommendation on routine imaging for patients with NLUTD. Yearly evaluation with a renal and bladder ultrasound and abdominal radiograph to evaluate for hydronephrosis and stone disease is considered adequate by neurourologists. Serum chemistry to evaluate kidney function is also helpful.

The Good Urodynamic Practice Guidelines recommend repeating UDS if "the initial test suggests an abnormality, leaves cause of troublesome lower urinary tract symptoms unresolved, or if there are technical problems preventing proper analysis."[35] If these guidelines were followed, all patients with NLUTD would need to undergo repeated studies. When determining how often a patient with NLUTD requires UDS, the urologist should be asking if a repeat UDS will change the patient's current bladder management. The European Association of Urology guidelines recommend following the International Continence Society urodynamics standards that state that UDS is "essential in following up the natural history of the disease or for checking the efficacy of treatment."[36,37] The American Urological Association guidelines have no specific recommendations regarding follow-up studies.[38]

There are various goals of treatment of patients with NLUTD, including[33]

- Upper urinary tract preservation or improvement
- Absence or control of infection
- Low storage pressures with adequate bladder capacity
- Low voiding pressures with adequate emptying ability if not performing intermittent catheterization

- Minimal or no incontinence
- Avoidance of indwelling catheter or stoma
- Social acceptability and adaptability of bladder management
- Vocational acceptability and adaptability of bladder management.

Keeping these goals in mind, the urologist should consider repeating UDS if the patient reports a change in bladder behavior or if routine studies, such as blood work, renal ultrasound, or other imaging, are abnormal.

What about the patients who are asymptomatic? The importance of UDS evaluation in this patient population is reflected in a retrospective study by Nosseir and colleagues.[39] They looked at 80 subjects with SCI who underwent UDS once a year for at least 5 consecutive years to determine how often treatment is modified based on UDS results. They defined treatment success as detrusor pressure less than 40 cm of water during filling and less than 90 cm of water during voiding, as well as absence of AD, less than three urinary tract infections per year, one continence pad per day, and no hydronephrosis or scarring on renal ultrasound. With a mean follow-up of 67.3 months, no subject had signs of renal damage and 77 of 80 (96%) subjects ultimately required treatment modification based on UDS findings during the study period. Of subjects who were symptomatic at time of UDS, all of them had abnormalities. More importantly, 68% of clinical failures would have been undetected based on symptoms alone.

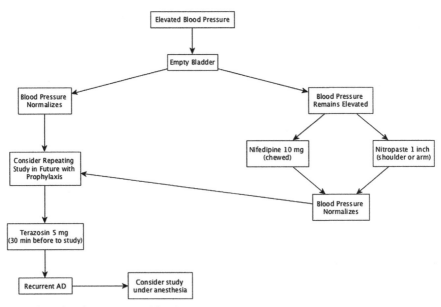

Fig. 3. Work-up algorithm for patients with NGB.

UDS can also be used to monitor patients before and after surgical interventions. Patients who have incontinence secondary to neurogenic detrusor activity require UDS to confirm the cause of incontinence before intravesical onabotulinumtoxinA injection. UDS may also be especially important for patients who reflex void and have undergone sphincterotomy. Failure of sphincterotomy has been defined as persistence of VUR or hydronephrosis, recurrent urinary tract infection, elevated postvoid residual volume, or persistent or recurrent AD. Light and colleagues[40] evaluated nine subjects who failed sphincterotomy and found that these subjects had low maximum intravesical pressures before voiding, suggesting detrusor hypocontractility. Long-term upper tract deterioration after sphincterotomy has been associated with DLPP greater than 40 cm of water,[41] suggesting that the initial sphincterotomy may need to be repeated. **Fig. 3** summarizes the initial work up and follow-up algorithm for patients with NGB.

Because UDS is time consuming, invasive, and has associated costs, attempts at using other clinical tools to assess a patient's need for UDS have been explored. Pannek and colleagues[42] looked at the use of detrusor wall thickness at various bladder volumes and its correlation to favorable UDS results and found that it was sensitive to determine the patients with no risk factors for renal damage; however, clinical parameters, such as detrusor overactivity and incontinence, could not be evaluated and may require further evaluation with UDS regardless of risk of renal damage.

SUMMARY

The main goal of management of a patient with NLUTD is to preserve renal function. UDS is the study of choice to identify patients at risk for upper tract deterioration as evidenced by high DLPP. This patient population presents a unique set of challenges because they often lack symptoms and/or the severity of symptoms does not correlate with the extent of potential risk to the kidneys. Patients with acute injury should have initial evaluation once bladder function returns, which often occurs around 3 months after injury. Children with spinal dysraphism should have initial studies performed early in life to identify those at higher risk. Follow-up UDS are performed in patients with change in symptoms, impairment of renal function, or concerning imaging studies.

REFERENCES

1. McGuire EJ. Urodynamics of the neurogenic bladder. Urol Clin North Am 2010;37(4):507–16.

2. Light K, Cinman A, Giles GR, et al. Urodynamics in congenital neurogenic bladder. S Afr J Surg 1978; 16(4):237–40.

3. McGuire EJ, Woodside JR, Borden TA, et al. Prognostic value of urodynamic testing in myelodysplastic patients. 1981. J Urol 2002;167(2 Pt 2):1049–53 [discussion: 1054].

4. Ghoniem GM, Bloom DA, McGuire EJ, et al. Bladder compliance in meningomyelocele children. J Urol 1989;141(6):1404–6.

5. Thomas D. Spinal cord injury. In: Mundy AR, Stephenson TP, Wein AJ, editors. Urodynamics: principals, practice and application. New York: Churchill Livingstone; 1984. p. 259–72.

6. Hald T, Bradley WE. Cystometry. In: Hald T, Bradely WE, editors. The urinary bladder: neurology and dynamics. Baltimore (MD): Williams & Wilkins; 1982. p. 110–7.

7. Abrams P. Urodynamics. 3rd edition. London: Springer-Verlag; 2006.

8. Palmer LS, Richards I, Kaplan WE. Age related bladder capacity and bladder capacity growth in children with myelomeningocele. J Urol 1997;158(3 Pt 2): 1261–4.

9. MacLellan DL, Bauer SB. Neuropathic dysfunction of the lower urinary tract. In: Wein AJ, Kavoussi LR, Novick AC, et al, editors. Campbell-Walsh urology, vol. 4, 10th edition. Philadelphia: Elsevier; 2012. p. 3431–56.

10. Joseph DB. The effect of medium-fill and slow-fill saline cystometry on detrusor pressure in infants and children with myelodysplasia. J Urol 1992; 147(2):444–6.

11. Barrett DM. Disposable (infant) surface electrocardiogram electrodes in urodynamics: a simultaneous comparative study of electrodes. J Urol 1980;124(5): 663–5.

12. Hilton J. Pain and therapeutic influence of mechanical physiological rest in accident and surgical disease. Lancet 1860;2:401.

13. Head H, Riddoch G. The autonomic bladder, excessive sweating, and some other reflex conditions in gross injuries of the spinal cord. Brain 1917;40:188.

14. Talaat M. Afferent impulses in nerves supplying the bladder. J Physiol 1938;32:121.

15. Guttman L, Whitteridge D. Effects of bladder distension on autonomic mechanisms after spinal cord injuries. Brain 1947;70:361.

16. Karlsson AK. Autonomic dysreflexia. Spinal Cord 1999;37(6):383–91.

17. Linsenmeyer TA, Campagnolo DI, Chou IH. Silent autonomic dysreflexia during voiding in men with spinal cord injuries. J Urol 1996;155(2):519–22.

18. Linsenmeyer TA, Bodner D, Creasey G. Bladder Management for Adults with Spinal Cord Injury: a clinical guideline for health-care providers.

In: Medicine CfSC, editor. Paralyzed Veterans of America; 2006.

19. Grossman E, Messerli FH, Grodzicki T, et al. Should a moratorium be placed on sublingual nifedipine capsules given for hypertensive emergencies and pseudoemergencies? JAMA 1996;276(16):1328–31.

20. Chancellor MB, Erhard MJ, Hirsch IH, et al. Prospective evaluation of terazosin for the treatment of autonomic dysreflexia. J Urol 1994;151(1):111–3.

21. Vaidyanathan S, Soni BM, Sett P, et al. Pathophysiology of autonomic dysreflexia: long-term treatment with terazosin in adult and paediatric spinal cord injury patients manifesting recurrent dysreflexic episodes. Spinal Cord 1998;36(11):761–70.

22. Dator DP, Hatchett L, Dyro FM, et al. Urodynamic dysfunction in walking myelodysplastic children. J Urol 1992;148(2 Pt 1):362–5.

23. Weld KJ, Dmochowski RR. Association of level of injury and bladder behavior in patients with post-traumatic spinal cord injury. Urology 2000;55(4):490–4.

24. Kaplan SA, Chancellor MB, Blaivas JG. Bladder and sphincter behavior in patients with spinal cord lesions. J Urol 1991;146(1):113–7.

25. Martin C, Salinas J, Fernandez-Duran A, et al. Genitourinary changes in multiple sclerosis: the need for a urodynamic study. Rev Neurol 2000;30(7):643–8 [in Spanish].

26. Gallien P, Robineau S, Nicolas B, et al. Vesicourethral dysfunction and urodynamic findings in multiple sclerosis: a study of 149 cases. Arch Phys Med Rehabil 1998;79(3):255–7.

27. Leu PB, Diokno AC. Epidemiology of the neurogenic bladder. In: Corcos J, Schick E, editors. (United Kingdom): Informa Healthcare; 2008.

28. Marinkovic SP, Badlani G. Voiding and sexual dysfunction after cerebrovascular accidents. J Urol 2001;165(2):359–70.

29. Ditunno JF, Little JW, Tessler A, et al. Spinal shock revisited: a four-phase model. Spinal Cord 2004; 42(7):383–95.

30. Sherrington CS. The integrative action of the nervous system. London: Constable & Company LTD; 1906.

31. Hall M. Synopsis of the diastaltic nervous system: or the system of the spinal marrow, and its reflex arcs; as the nervous agent in all the functions of ingestion and of egestion in the animal oeconomy. London: Mallett J; 1850.

32. Thomas D, O'Flynn KJ. Spinal cord injury. In: Mundy AR, Stephenson T, Wein AJ, editors. Urodynamics: principles, practice and application. 2nd edition. London: Churchill Livingstone; 1994. p. 345–58.

33. Wein AJ, Dmochowski RR. Neuromuscular dysfunction of the lower urinary tract. In: Wein AJ, Kavoussi LR, Novick AC, editors. Campbell-Walsh urology, vol. 3, 10th edition. Philadelphia: WB Saunders; 2012. p. 1909–46.

34. Hosker G, Rosier P, Gajewski J, editors. Dynamic testing. International Consultation on Incontinence. (United Kingdom): Health Publications; 2009.

35. Schafer W, Abrams P, Liao L, et al. Good urodynamic practices: uroflowmetry, filling cystometry, and pressure-flow studies. Neurourol Urodyn 2002; 21(3):261–74.

36. Stohrer M, Blok B, Castro-Diaz D, et al. EAU guidelines on neurogenic lower urinary tract dysfunction. Eur Urol 2009;56(1):81–8.

37. Homma Y, editor. Urodynamics. 2nd International Consultation on Incontinence; 2002 July 1–3, 2001. Paris: Plymbridge Distributors, Ltd; 2002.

38. Winters JC, Dmochowski RR, Goldman HB, et al. Urodynamic studies in adults: AUA/SUFU guideline. J Urol 2012;188(Suppl 6):2464–72.

39. Nosseir M, Hinkel A, Pannek J. Clinical usefulness of urodynamic assessment for maintenance of bladder function in patients with spinal cord injury. Neurourol Urodyn 2007;26(2):228–33.

40. Light JK, Beric A, Wise PG. Predictive criteria for failed sphincterotomy in spinal cord injury patients. J Urol 1987;138(5):1201–4.

41. Kim YH, Kattan MW, Boone TB. Bladder leak point pressure: the measure for sphincterotomy success in spinal cord injured patients with external detrusor-sphincter dyssynergia. J Urol 1998;159(2): 493–6 [discussion: 496–7].

42. Pannek J, Bartel P, Gocking K, et al. Clinical usefulness of ultrasound assessment of detrusor wall thickness in patients with neurogenic lower urinary tract dysfunction due to spinal cord injury: urodynamics made easy? World J Urol 2013;31(3): 659–64.

Pressure Flow Studies in Men and Women

Sylvester E. Onyishi, MD, Christian O. Twiss, MD*

KEYWORDS

• Urodynamics • Pressure flow study • Urinary obstruction • Detrusor underactivity

KEY POINTS

- There are well-established pressure flow criteria for urinary obstruction in men.
- The pressure flow criteria for female urinary obstruction are not well established because of differences in female voiding dynamics compared with men; typically, other information such as radiographic data and clinical symptoms are needed to facilitate the diagnosis.
- Detrusor underactivity remains a poorly studied clinical condition without definitive urodynamic diagnostic criteria.

INTRODUCTION

Pressure flow urodynamics study is a well-established diagnostic tool for evaluating bladder outlet obstruction in men. Nomograms such as the Abrams-Griffiths nomogram, the Passive Urethral Resistance Relation, and the ICS nomogram have been established and accepted for use in male voiding dysfunction. Parameters obtained from these nomograms, such as the Bladder Outlet Obstruction Index (BOOI), Qmax (maximum flow), and PdetQmax (detrusor pressure at maximum flow), have accepted cutoff values for defining bladder outlet obstruction (BOO) in men with benign prostatic hyperplasia (BPH) due to the high prevalence of BPH and the associated symptoms. Because of differences in the anatomy of lower urinary tract and voiding dynamics between the sexes, established criteria for urodynamic obstruction in men do not apply to women, and there are currently no widely accepted cutoff values for defining BOO in women.

Another cause of lower urinary tract symptoms (LUTS) that cannot be distinguished from BOO purely based on symptoms and uroflow study is detrusor underactvity (DU). Although this is not as prevalent in men as BOO, it accounts for a significant proportion of men with LUTS and is common in women with urinary retention.[1] According to the International Continence Society (ICS), DU is defined as a detrusor contraction of inadequate magnitude and/or duration to effect complete bladder emptying in the absence of urethral obstruction.[2] DU may arise de novo and coexist with BOO, and it can be a complication of longstanding untreated BOO. DU can only be diagnosed via pressure flow studies.

In this report, we strive to highlight the role of pressure flow studies (PFS) in diagnosis of BOO and DU and determine what is known about the urodynamic criteria to diagnose these conditions in men and women.

BASICS OF PFS

PFS are the essential urodynamic studies used to evaluate the voiding or emptying characteristics of the lower urinary tract by monitoring the detrusor pressure and uroflow simultaneously. Detrusor contractility and bladder outlet resistance are the 2 main parameters determined from PFS. Three

Funding: None.
Disclosures: None.
Division of Urology, University of Arizona College of Medicine, PO Box 245077, 1501 North Campbell Avenue, Tucson, AZ 85724, USA
* Corresponding author.
E-mail address: ctwiss@surgery.arizona.edu

Urol Clin N Am 41 (2014) 453–467
http://dx.doi.org/10.1016/j.ucl.2014.04.007
0094-0143/14/$ – see front matter © 2014 Elsevier Inc. All rights reserved.

urologic.theclinics.com

fundamental voiding states may be identified in PFS:

1. Low detrusor pressure and high flow rate, which signifies the unobstructed state
2. High detrusor pressure and low flow rate, which signifies the obstructed state
3. Low detrusor pressure and low flow rate, which is indicative of detrusor underactivity

It is important to note that borderline cases with coexistence of obstruction and impaired contractility are possible and that the above classifications are not absolute. The nomograms described below have been devised to interpret PFS based on the plot of the detrusor pressure at maximum urinary flow (PdetQmax) versus the maximum urinary flow rate (Qmax). Typical unobstructed and obstructed PFS are shown in **Fig. 1**.[3] Intravesical and abdominal pressures are measured using catheters with pressure transducer, whereas the detrusor pressure is calculated by subtracting the abdominal pressure from the intravesical pressure.

MEASURING URODYNAMIC OBSTRUCTION
PFS in Men

In men, Qmax of less than 10 has been used as the cutoff to suggest obstruction.[4] About 90% of men with a Qmax less than 10 have obstruction.[4] On the other hand, 25% to 30% of men with decreased flow rate do not have obstruction.[4] Thus, decreased flow rate by itself is not sufficient to accurately diagnose outlet resistance, as it may be indicative of obstruction, impaired bladder contractility, or a combination of both. Simultaneous measurement of detrusor pressure and flow rate during voiding helps distinguish the causes of reduced flow rate by simultaneously assessing detrusor and outlet function as they relate to voiding.

To this end, several well-established nomograms and concepts have been advanced to categorize the voiding pattern in men as obstructed, equivocal, or unobstructed. These are (1) the Abrams-Griffiths nomogram, (2) the Urethral Resistance Factor (URA), (3) the Passive Urethral Resistance Relation (PURR), and (4) the Linear Passive Urethral Resistance Relation (LinPURR).[5–8]

The Abrams-Griffiths Nomogram

The data for the Abrams-Griffiths nomogram (**Fig. 2**) were originally obtained via PFS of 117 men age 55 and older evaluated for possible BPH.[8,9] By plotting PdetQmax on Y axis and Qmax on X axis, 3 zones are generated, representing obstructed, unobstructed, and equivocal micturition. The boundaries for the zones were created by a combination of theoretical and empiric observations. Specifically, patients were classified clinically as obstructed or unobstructed based on clinical criteria established in the earlier work of Abrams and colleagues[10–12] before undergoing pressure flow studies. In addition, the pressure flow plots were represented as obstructed or unobstructed based on separate sets of empiric criteria previously established by Bates and colleagues[13] and Griffiths.[14] The nomogram was then constructed by comparing the 2 methods of assessment, clinically and from pressure flow plots.

This nomogram has been used in studying the outcome of prostatectomy performed for BOO. Jensen and colleagues[15] noted significant improvement in pressure flow parameters after prostatectomy in obstructed patients but not in unobstructed patients using this nomogram. The improvements in pressure flow parameters were noted to correlate with subjective improvement in LUTS. Other investigators subsequently duplicated these findings.[9,16] Thus, the utility of the nomogram is primarily in making an accurate diagnosis of male BOO and identifying patients who are likely to benefit from surgical intervention.

One of the early criticisms of the Abrams-Griffiths nomogram was the lack of a quantitative measure of obstruction. This eventually led to the formulation of the Abrams-Griffiths (AG) number from this nomogram. The Abrams-Griffiths nomogram and the AG number form the basis of the ICS nomogram as discussed later. Another issue is that the Abrams-Griffiths nomogram by its nature does not permit the diagnosis of impaired contractility with or without coexisting BOO.

The Concept of the Urethral Resistance Factor

In a separate work, Griffiths and colleagues[17] derived a single parameter called *urethral resistance factor* (URA) for quantifying urethral resistance. This was derived from the pressure flow plots of men with obstruction caused by BPH. This model was largely based on the conceptualization of the urethra as an active tube with an effective cross-sectional area. Flow is initiated in such a tube once the minimum pressure, termed *urethral opening pressure* (Puo) is reached or slightly exceeded. Once Puo is reached, voiding occurs, assuming that the urethra remains relaxed during voiding. Based on this concept, the authors generated a series of curves of constant resistance (**Fig. 3**) and noted that these closely follow the pressure flow plots under relaxed conditions.

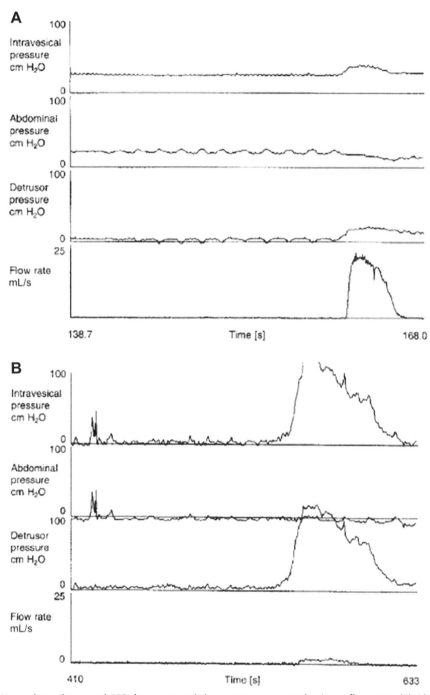

Fig. 1. (*A*) Normal, unobstructed PFS shows normal detrusor pressure and urinary flow rate. (*B*) Obstructed PFS shows classic high detrusor pressure and low urinary flow rate. (*From* Griffiths D. Basics of pressure-flow studies. World J Urol 1995;13:31; with permission.)

Any pair of pressure-flow (PQ) values occurring during micturition can thus be represented by a point on this graph and the value of the Puo for the curve on which the point lies represents the URA, expressed in cm H_2O. The authors also showed that URA can be calculated with the Equation 1, which will give a valid number for URA even if the PQ plot does not follow the ideal form as depicted in **Fig. 3** as long as Qmax and corresponding PdetQmax are known.

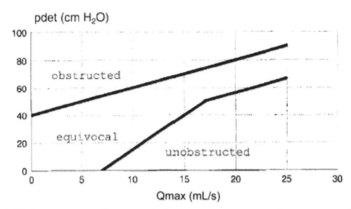

Fig. 2. The Abrams-Griffiths nomogram. The Y-axis is detrusor pressure at maximum urinary flow (PdetQmax) and the X-axis is maximum urinary flow (Qmax). (*From* Lim CS, Abrams P. The Abrams-Griffith nomogram. World J Urol 1995;13:35; with permission.)

$$URA = P_{uo} = \frac{\left[(1 + 4dQ^2Pdet)^{\frac{1}{2}} - 1 \right]}{2dQ^2} \quad (1)$$

where Q is the flow rate, $Pdet$ is detrusor pressure, Puo the urethral opening pressure, and d is a constant related to cross-sectional area, c, of the urethra ($d = Puo^2/c$ and has a value of 3.8×10^{-4})

Griffiths and colleagues[17] noted that it is not easy to define a single urethral resistance parameter universally applicable to all groups (adults and children) because of the difference in the causes and locations of obstruction among different groups of patients. For instance, in men, the etiology of outlet obstruction is most commonly BPH, but in women, outlet obstruction is uncommon and, when present, is typically both iatrogenic in nature and located proximally. In children, obstructions tend to be distal, such as meatal stenosis, and the PQ plots tend to be constrictive in nature versus compressive in adults. Thus, URA derived for adults may not be valid in children. The authors concluded that URA is better used for a specific group of patients with similar etiology of obstruction, in this case BPH, although the above equation was also noted to be a close approximation for cases of

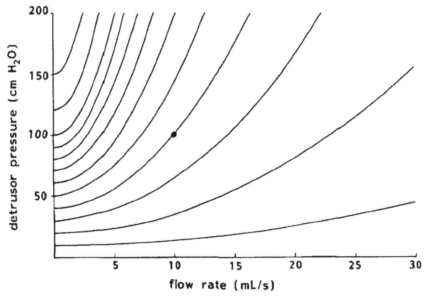

Fig. 3. Pressure/flow curves for various constant values of URA from 10 to 150 cm H_2O. The filled circle represents a moment of voiding when detrusor pressure is 100 cm H_2O, and the urine flow rate is 10 mL/s. This point lies on the curve for URA of 40 cm H_2O. (*From* Griffiths D, Mastrigt RV, Bosch R. Quantification of Urethral resistance and bladder function during voiding, with special reference to the effects of prostate size reduction on urethral obstruction due to benign prostatic hyperplasia. Neurourol Urodyn 1989;8:20; with permission.)

obstruction in adult women.[17] The URA cutoff value for obstruction is 29 and greater.

Lim and Abrams[9] showed that the AG number and URA correlate quite well in the diagnosis of obstruction caused by BPH as depicted in the scatter diagram in **Fig. 4**. The data for comparison were obtained by calculating both the AG number and URA for pre- and post-prostatectomy pressure-flow data in 85 patients with BPH. The Pearson correlation coefficient for the 2 factors is 0.9, which is an indication of good agreement between the 2 methods of assessment. The correlation is much better at lower grades of obstruction and in the unobstructed zones.

Passive Urethral Resistance Relation

In deriving the passive urethral resistance relation (PURR) curve (**Fig. 5**), the flow dynamics in the urethra/bladder outlet were modeled as flow in a distensible and collapsible tube in a perfectly relaxed condition. Similar to modeling the URA as discussed above, flow is also initiated in this model once the urethral opening pressure, Puo, is reached. The PURR is fundamentally based on the concept of the urethral resistance relation (URR) proposed by Griffiths.[7,14,18,19] This concept suggests that flow is initiated when intrinsic bladder pressure equals intrinsic urethral pressure, and the rate of flow increases sharply with further increases in intrinsic bladder pressure. Thus, the curve obtained by plotting Pdet versus Q during the course of a micturition event represents urethral resistance to flow, independent of detrusor function.

In an ideal condition, once flow is initiated, the flow rate increases, and the maximum flow rate is established in accordance with the maximum voiding pressure. Also, in this ideal condition, the outlet pressure near the end of voiding is same as that in the beginning. In addition to the Puo, the other critical parameter that governs the outflow condition in a perfectly relaxed bladder outlet is the effective cross-sectional area of the flow controlling zone, which, according to Schafer[7,19] is close to the genitourinary diaphragm. When there is an obstruction, however, the obstruction itself takes over the role of the flow controlling zone. Using these 2 parameters (ie, Puo reflecting the collapsible nature of the tube and, A, the effective cross sectional area) normal pressure/flow curves were fit to Equation 2 to obtain the PURR curve as shown in **Fig. 6**.[19]

$$P_{det} = P_{uo} + \frac{1}{c} Q^2 \qquad (2)$$

where c = a constant = $2A^2$

Other inherent assumptions made in deriving this curve are that flow is steady through a constant cross-sectional area and that fluid viscosity and other energy losses are negligible. Based on the underlying model, PURR essentially describes the impact of a passive bladder outlet on voiding independent of bladder function.

Schafer[7] noted that the ideal PURR curve sometimes deviated from normal PQ data in clinical voiding studies mainly because of variations in bladder outlet properties assumed to be constant in the ideal PURR. For instance, the opening pressure at the start of voiding tends to be higher than the pressure at the termination of voiding (recall that these were assumed to be the same in ideal situations). This deviation was noted to be related to the passive, viscoelastic relaxation of the outlet

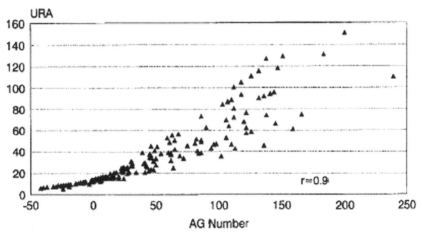

Fig. 4. Scatter diagram of AG number versus URA. The Pearson correlation coefficient for the 2 factors is 0.9, which denotes good correlation between AG number and URA. (*From* Lim CS, Abrams P. The Abrams-Griffith nomogram. World J Urol 1995;13:37; with permission.)

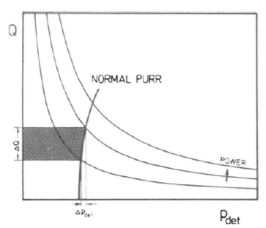

Fig. 5. The normal PURR, as described in men, defines the potential relationship between pressure and flow rate determined by the bladder outlet. Lines of constant power representative of detrusor strength appear as hyperbolae. (*From* Schafer W. The contribution of the bladder outlet to the relation between pressure and flow rate during micturition. In: Hinman F Jr, Boyarsky S, editors. Benign prostatic hypertrophy. New York: Springer-Verlag; 1983. p. 480; with permission.)

tissues during distension. In addition, contraction of external sphincter may actively change the outflow conditions by decreasing the effective cross-sectional area or increasing the opening pressure and as such lead to a deviation from the ideal. This is especially true in a case of severe dyssynergic or dysfunctional voiding in which the actual passive state of the outlet may not even be reached.

The PURR curves for obstructive BPH and urethral stricture disease (see **Fig. 6**) have been described, and the review of PURR curves for these two scenarios of obstruction greatly facilitates the understanding of the concepts of urethral opening pressure and the urethral flow-controlling zone (region of lowest cross-sectional area) as they relate to voiding. In obstruction caused by BPH, the PURR is described as compressive and is shifted to the right, reflecting the increased opening pressure required to initiate voiding as the major process. In other words, the urethral wall exhibits reduced distensibility in BPH compared with the normal condition and, as such, higher pressure is required to open the urethra and initiate urinary flow. Once flow starts, however, further increases in pressure result in increases in flow. In stricture disease, the curve is described as constrictive and appears flat. The flat nature is deemed to be related to the decrease in the effective cross-sectional area of the flow-controlling zone. In this scenario, increases in

pressure fail to result in significant increases in flow because of the reduced urethral cross-sectional area. In general, the PURR by position and slope provides information about opening pressure, which is a reflection of the degree of compressive obstruction and the effective lumen size of the flow rate controlling zone, which is a measure of degree of constrictive obstruction.[7,19,20]

Linear Passive Urethral Resistance Relation

The nomograms and the tools for analyzing micturition described thus far focus on the assessment of the bladder outlet. The linear passive urethral resistance relation (LinPURR) fully integrates the function of the detrusor and bladder outlet in describing the dynamics of micturition. To this end, the LinPURR was derived as a modified version of the PURR with straight lines instead of parabolic curves.[18,21]

Conceptually, the detrusor can be described as a source of mechanical power for voiding and the bladder outlet as the physical entity that dissipates this power in the form of flow rate and pressure during voiding.[18] The detrusor power is proportional to the filling volume of the bladder or, more precisely, the prestretched length of the detrusor muscle. Additionally, both detrusor pressure and urinary flow rate are expressions of detrusor power that have an inverse relationship. In other words, for a certain power generated by detrusor, which is dissipated by the bladder outlet in the form of flow rate and pressure, a high flow rate implies a low pressure and vice versa, as the product of the two must necessarily be constant. Based on this concept, a series of hyperbolic curves representing the contractile capabilities of the detrusor for certain activation are superimposed on parabolic curves similar to PURR curves representing the specific outflow condition.

A linearized version of detrusor strength was derived and superimposed on the linear PURR for a composite graph that can be used to analyze voiding in terms of integrated detrusor and outlet function. Specifically, the two critical parameters used to construct the linear PURR are the opening pressure, Puo, which, as described previously, is the lowest detrusor pressure at which flow starts or stops, and the pressure at maximum flow rate, PdetQmax. A straight line connecting these two points on a pressure flow graph represents a simple linear PURR, from which specific characterization of the individual outflow conditions during a single voiding event can be obtained. Several such points are plotted and different grades of obstruction delineated based on an indirect

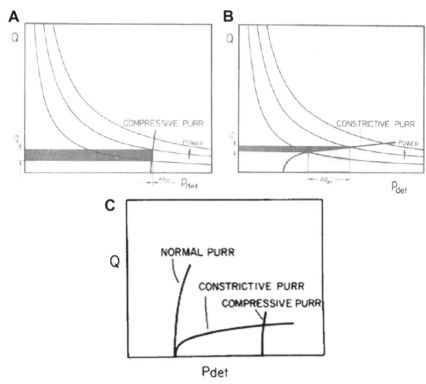

Fig. 6. (*A*) The compressive PURR, typically found in prostatic obstruction, is characterized by higher opening pressure without major changes in the slope. (*B*) The constrictive PURR results from a decrease in the effective cross-sectional area, as reflected in the flat shape, without an increase in the normal opening pressure. This is typical for anterior urethral strictures. Flow rate changes little with increased detrusor power after the initial steep increase. (*C*) Comparison of normal, constrictive, and compressive PURR: notice that the slope of normal PURR is similar to compressive PURR, although compressive PURR is shifted to the right, reflecting the increase in the opening pressure, Puo. Normal PURR and constrictive PURR have similar opening pressures, but the curve of constrictive PURR is flat, reflecting decrease in effective cross-sectional area of the urethral flow controlling zone. (*From* [*A, B*] Schafer W. The contribution of the bladder outlet to the relation between pressure and flow rate during micturition. In: Hinman F Jr, Boyarsky S, editors. Benign prostatic hypertrophy. New York: Springer-Verlag; 1983. p. 482, with permission; and [*C*] Blavais J. Multichannel urodynamics studies. Urology 1984;23(5):425, with permission.)

approach from computerized analysis of a database of more than 2000 voiding studies with the PURR, **Fig. 7.**[18]

The LinPURR curve was divided into 7 zones (0–VI) corresponding to increasing grades of obstruction, that is, zones 0 to I (unobstructed), zone II (equivocal or mild obstruction), and zones III to VI (more severe grades of obstruction). The borderlines for the grading schemes were defined based on the Puo. It was suggested[18] that such a detailed grading scheme (7 zones) would provide more meaningful information in the assessment of minor changes in outflow conditions as may be expected in drug trials compared with simpler classification schemes. This can be viewed as both a strength and a drawback because of the greater complexity involved compared with other nomograms.

Linear grading of detrusor strength or contractility is also implemented. It is categorized as strong, normal, weak, and very weak. It was noted that grading of detrusor strength is less reproducible compared with the outlet function in this model.[18]

The ICS Nomogram

In 1995, Lim and Abrams[9] noted that patients were identically classified by the Abrams-Griffiths nomogram and the LinPURR when compared.[4] The Abrams-Griffiths nomogram and the Urethral Resistance Factor also showed about 94% agreement in classifying degree of obstruction.[9,17] It was noted that when the Abrams-Griffiths nomogram is superimposed on the LinPURR curve, the line separating the obstructed zone from equivocal zone in the Abrams-Griffiths nomogram

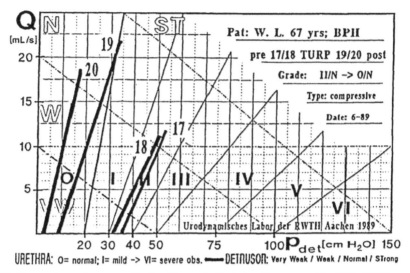

Fig. 7. LinPURR. Figure shows how a patient with grade 2 obstruction caused by BPH (17/18 pre-TURP on the graph), was reclassified to grade 0 (19/20) post-TURP. Notice the 7 zones for grading obstruction and the 4 zones for grading detrusor contraction. (*From* Schafer W. Principle and clinical application of advanced urodynamic analysis of voiding function. Urol Clin North Am 1990;17:563; with permission.)

is equivalent to the line separating zone II from zone III on the LinPURR, which represents obstructed and slightly obstructed, respectively (**Fig. 8**). This observation is significant given the relative simplicity of the Abrams-Griffiths nomogram compared with the more complex LinPURR.

Lim and Abrams proceeded to derive the AG number from the equation of the line dividing the obstructed from the equivocal range in the Abrams-Griffiths nomogram. The Equation 3 is represented as:

$$AG\ number = Pdet@Qmax - 2(Qmax) \qquad (3)$$

where 2 is the gradient or slope of this line

This line intercepts the pressure axis of the Abrams-Griffiths nomogram at 40 cm H_2O. Therefore, points in the obstructed zone will have AG numbers greater than 40, whereas points in the

equivocal and unobstructed zones will have AG numbers less than 40. By applying the same principle to the line separating the equivocal from the unobstructed zone, they concluded that most patients with AG number less than 15 are unobstructed, whereas those with AG numbers 15 to 40 are equivocal (**Fig. 9**).[9] In 1997, the provisional ICS recommendations adopted the equation for the AG number as standard for use in men with LUTS suggestive of BPH and has since renamed it the *Bladder Outlet Obstruction Index* (BOOI). This subsequently became the basis for the ICS nomogram (**Fig. 10**), and the cut off values were established as follows: BOOI greater than 40, obstructed; BOOI 20 to 40, equivocal; and BOOI less than 20, unobstructed.[2]

The ICS nomogram with BOOI is a useful tool for the evaluation of patients with suspected bladder

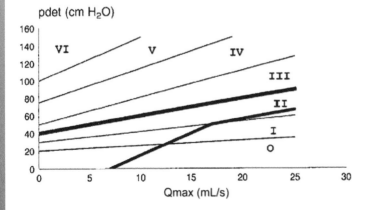

Fig. 8. The LinPURR superimposed on the Abrams-Griffiths nomogram. The boundary between zones 2 and 3 of the LinPURR is the same as the boundary between the obstructed and equivocal zone in the Abrams-Griffiths nomogram. (*From* Lim CS, Abrams P. The Abrams-Griffith nomogram. World J Urol 1995;13:38; with permission.)

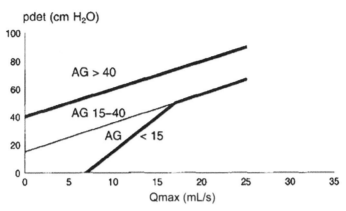

Fig. 9. The AG number. AG greater than 40, obstructed; AG of 15 to 40, equivocal; AG less than 15, majority un-obstructed. (*From* Lim CS, Abrams P. The Abrams-Griffith nomogram. World J Urol 1995;13:36; with permission.)

outlet obstruction, especially when it clearly indicates obstruction or no obstruction. However, when patients fall into the equivocal range on the ICS nomogram, frequently other sources of information such as clinical symptom severity and response to therapeutic interventions are required to assist in treatment decision making.

PFS in Women

Parameters from PFS have been used to establish acceptable nomograms for men as outlined above. However, these nomograms are not applicable to women for several reasons. First, because of anatomic differences, the voiding dynamics differ significantly between men and women. Women typically void at lower detrusor pressures than men. Some women are able to void to completion by simply relaxing the pelvic floor musculature while others augment voiding by abdominal straining (valsalva voiding).[22,23] In addition, the nomograms in men were established by extensively studying men with BPH, which is a highly prevalent condition. There is no equivalent prevalent condition consistently causing bladder outlet obstruction in women as BPH does in

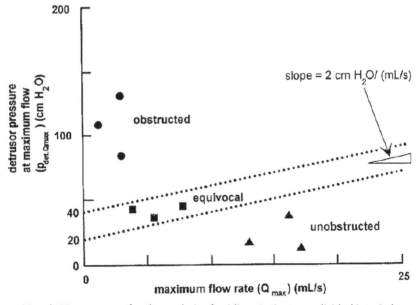

Fig. 10. The provisional ICS nomogram for the analysis of voiding. Patients are divided into 3 classes according to the BOOI (BOOI = PdetQmax − 2 Qmax). Obstructed (BOOI≥40); Equivocal (BOOI = 20–40); Unobstructed (BOOI≤20). (*From* Griffiths D, Hofner K, van Magstrigt R, et al. Standardization of terminology of lower urinary tract function: pressure-flow studies of voiding, urethral resistance and urethral obstruction. Neurourol Urodyn 1997;16:10; with permission.)

men. The estimated prevalence of bladder outlet obstruction in women ranges between 2.7% and 23%.[24–28] Some of the known causes of obstruction in women include dysfunctional voiding, primary bladder neck obstruction, uterovaginal prolapse, and complications of incontinence surgery.[29] Attempts have been made to establish a standard for the diagnosis of BOO in women, and all can be grouped into 1 of 3 categories: (1) pressure flow cutoff criteria, (2) videourodynamics, and (3) nomograms. Although differences exist in both sexes with regard to pressure flow parameters that define outlet obstruction, the concept of high pressure, low flow voiding as the fundamental definition of outlet obstruction remains the same.

Pressure flow cutoff values of Qmax less than 11 to 15 mL/sec and PdetQmax greater than 20 to 25 have been established by several authors as diagnostic of female BOO using different study populations and control groups.[30–33] Another cutoff criterion proposed by Cormier and colleagues[34] is the use of the area under the curve of detrusor pressure during voiding adjusted for voided volume. They performed linear discriminant analysis using traditional classification (obstructed, equivocal, and unobstructed) based on clinical evaluation and pressure flow study data. The area under the curve of detrusor pressure adjusted for volume (AUCdet/vol) of 5.83 cm water/sec/mL separated the obstructed from equivocal cases, whereas AUCdet/vol of 2.56 cm water/sec/mL separated the equivocal from unobstructed cases. The agreement between these cutoff values based on linear discriminant analysis using AUCdet/vol and traditional classification was noted to be 86%, 36%, and 57% in cases of unobstructed, equivocal, and obstructed, respectively.[34]

Nitti and colleagues[29] utilized radiographic evidence of obstruction on videourodynamic evaluation to assist in the diagnosis of female BOO. Their work involved a retrospective chart review of 261 women with nonneurogenic voiding dysfunction. They argued that obstruction may be missed in some women if strict criteria of high pressure low flow voiding are used, as women typically void at lower detrusor pressures than men. Patients were classified as obstructed if there was radiographic evidence of a closed or narrow bladder neck during voiding or a discrete area of narrowing in the urethra associated with proximal dilation in the presence of sustained detrusor contraction of any magnitude with reduced or delayed urinary flow rate. When urodynamic parameters were compared, the obstructed cases had significantly higher mean PdetQmax (42.8 vs 22.1 cm H_2O), lower mean Qmax (9 vs 20.2 mL/s), and higher mean postvoid residual (157 vs 33 mL) than

unobstructed cases. However, there was a wide range of values for these parameters as reflected in the standard deviation.[29] Given the wide range of values observed, the authors proposed that strict cutoff values defining obstruction would lack specificity.

In 2000, Blavais and Groutz[24] and Mahfouz and colleagues,[35] proposed a nomogram for defining bladder outlet obstruction by reviewing a urodynamics database of 600 women. In constructing the nomogram, they used two parameters: free Qmax (free flow or noninvasive flow rate) instead of Qmax (invasive or pressure flow study) and Pdetmax (maximum detrusor pressure during voiding) instead of PdetQmax (detrusor pressure at maximum flow). This was due to the difficulty in performing uroflowmetry in women with the catheter in place, as the presence of a catheter tends to affect the urinary flow rate. Pdetmax was preferred over PdetQmax because (1) they found no statistically significant difference between the two and (2) PdetQmax cannot be plotted in cases of urinary retention because there is no measurable flow (despite the possible presence of a detrusor contraction). The criteria for defining BOO included one or more of the following: (1) free Qmax $\leq$12 mL/s in repeated free flow studies combined with sustained detrusor contraction and PdetQmax $\geq$20 cm H_2O in pressure flow study; (2) obvious radiographic evidence of bladder outlet obstruction in the presence of a sustained detrusor contraction of at least 20 cm H_2O; or (3) inability to void with transurethral catheter in place despite sustained detrusor contraction of at least 20 cm H_2O.

Using cluster analysis, three clusters of free Qmax/Pdetmax plot were identified (**Fig. 11**): (1) low pressure/high flow, (2) high pressure/low flow, and (3) low-to-intermediate pressure/flow values. The low-to-intermediate pressure/flow cluster was subdivided into two categories, and together with the other clusters, a 4-zone nomogram was developed (**Fig. 12**). Using this nomogram, the authors noted that all of the obstructed women were correctly classified as obstructed and further subclassified as mildly obstructed (68%), moderately obstructed (24%), and severely obstructed (8%). They found a positive correlation between subjective severity of symptoms (assessed by American Urological Association Symptom Score) and the nomogram zones. Of the patients classified as unobstructed, the nomogram correctly identified 80% as unobstructed, 8% as mildly obstructed, and 12% on the borderline between no obstruction and mild obstruction.

This nomogram is a helpful tool in the diagnosis of female obstruction, but because of the

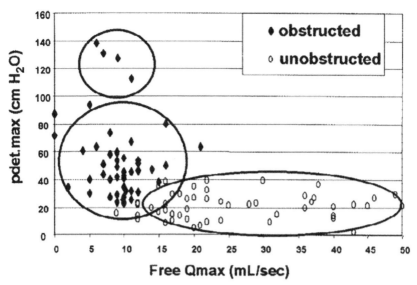

Fig. 11. Distributions of free Qmax versus Pdetmax plot according to clinical diagnosis. (*From* Blavais JG, Groutz A. Bladder outlet obstruction nomogram for women with lower urinary tract symptomatology. Neurourol Urodyn 2000;19:559; with permission.)

variability in female voiding dynamics, the diagnosis of female BOO remains difficult and often involves consideration of clinical, urodynamic, and radiographic data to make the final assessment. Additionally, the outcomes for surgical intervention (eg, transurethral resection of the prostate or simple open prostatectomy) to treat obstruction in men are linked to a urodynamic diagnosis of obstruction,[9,15,16] whereas there is a lack of similar such evidence in women undergoing surgical intervention for obstruction (eg, urethrolysis).[36]

MEASURING DETRUSOR UNDERACTIVITY

DU remains an understudied clinical condition, and the understanding of the pathophysiology, diagnosis, and treatment remains rudimentary as documented in the 2010 International Consultation on Incontinence Research Society meeting.[37] About 10% to 20% of men with low flow have DU[38–40] yet a Medline search for publications between the year 1980 and 2010 using the terms *detrusor underactivity* and *underactive bladder* yielded only 93 and 80 publications, respectively,

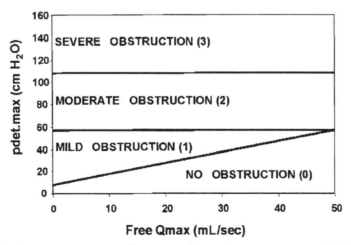

Fig. 12. Bladder outlet obstruction nomogram for women. (*From* Blavais JG, Groutz A. Bladder outlet obstruction nomogram for women with lower urinary tract symptomatology. Neurourol Urodyn 2000;19:561; with permission.)

in the last 30 years.[37] This is in stark contrast to a similar search using the terms *detrusor overactivity* and *overactive bladder*, which yielded 1223 and 2688 hits, respectively, within the same timeframe. Clearly, more emphasis has been placed on outlet function than bladder function during voiding.

The pathophysiologic mechanism underlying DU secondary to long-standing BPH is believed to be owing to loss of detrusor muscle cells, collagen deposition, and axonal degeneration seen in the decompensation phase of the bladder in BOO caused by BPH.[1,41–43] Other etiologies of DU include diabetes mellitus, neurologic problems involving the lumbosacral nerves, chronic UTI, and anticholinergic medications.

The importance of proper diagnosis and distinction between BOO and DU is underscored by the finding that surgical intervention geared toward relieving obstruction caused by BPH does not provide lasting symptomatic relief of LUTS when the underlying etiology is in fact DU and not BOO.[44] In addition to the LinPURR discussed above, two other measures based on computer-urodynamic investigation and quantification of detrusor pressure during voiding have been suggested to quantify detrusor power or contractility. These are the (1) Griffiths Power (Watt) Factor and (2) the Bladder Contractility Index, which are discussed below.

The Power (Watt) Factor

Based on the concept of the Hill equation, which governs the fundamental relationship between the force of contraction and the speed of shortening of a contracting muscle, the strength of detrusor contraction may be expressed in terms of a combination of the detrusor pressure, flow rate, and bladder volume.[17,45] These parameters are used to calculate the Power (Watt) Factor, abbreviated WF. This is considered representative of the mechanical power developed by the contracting bladder or, alternatively, an estimate of the isovolumetric detrusor pressure that would develop if voiding were interrupted. The equations and derivation of the WF are beyond the scope of this report.

WF varies during the entire course of voiding, and a representative value such as its maximum value (WFmax) or the value at maximum flow may be used to describe detrusor strength for a single micturition event. However, it remains controversial whether WFmax or value at maximum flow provides a better estimate of detrusor strength for clinical application.[37] In addition, there is no widely accepted threshold value of WF for defining DU, although expert opinion suggests a WFmax of 7.0 W/m^2 may be used as a possible threshold.[37]

Bladder Contraction Index and the Composite Nomogram

As previously noted in the LinPURR nomogram (see **Fig. 7**), bladder contractility can be categorized into 4 groups: strong, normal, weak, and very weak. The slope of the lines separating these categories is given by the formula in Equation 4. Because these lines are parallel to each other, they have the same slope.[4,46] This formula describing the slope subsequently came to be known as the *bladder contraction index* (BCI).

$$BCI = Pdet\ Qmax + 5\ Qmax \qquad (4)$$

The intersections of these lines on the pressure axis of the LinPURR define the boundaries for the contractility groups; thus, BCI greater than 150 is considered strong contractility, 100 to 150 constitute normal contractility, and values less than 100 are considered weak contractility (**Fig. 13**). Both BCI and BOOI can be calculated from the corresponding formulas (Equations 3 and 4) with or without nomograms and can be combined to

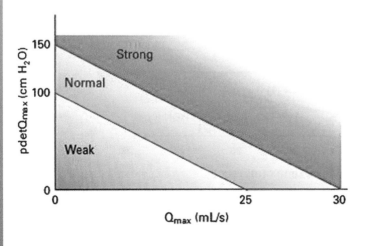

Fig. 13. The Bladder contractility index (BCI) divides patients into 3 categories: strong (BCI≥150), normal (BCI = 100–150), and weak (BCI≤100). (*From* Abrams P. Bladder outlet obstruction index, bladder contractility index and bladder voiding efficiency: three simple indices to define bladder voiding function. BJU Int 1999;84:15; with permission.)

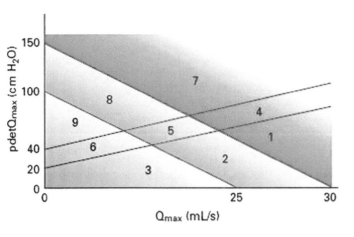

Fig. 14. A composite nomogram allowing categorization of patients into 9 zones based on BOOI and BCI. For instance, zone 1 represents patients with strong contractility and no obstruction, whereas zone 9 represents patients with weak contractility and obstruction. (*From* Abrams P. Bladder outlet obstruction index, bladder contractility index and bladder voiding efficiency: three simple indices to define bladder voiding function. BJU Int 1999;84:15; with permission.)

categorize any group of men into 9 classes by combining the 3 obstruction categories and the 3 contractility categories. The resulting spectrum of contractility and obstruction ranges from group 1 (no obstruction and good contractility) to group 9 (obstruction with weak contractility) (**Fig. 14**).[46]

All the concepts for measuring and classifying detrusor underactivity were developed for adult men and not validated in women. It is also unclear whether they equally describe bladder power. No clear threshold values for defining detrusor underactivity have been established at this time.

SUMMARY

Clearly established pressure flow criteria exist for men that are useful in categorizing and assisting in decision making for male voiding dysfunction caused by obstruction. This report reviewed the various concepts and nomograms that ultimately contributed to the development of the ICS nomogram, which is widely used to evaluate male urinary obstruction.

Similar pressure flow criteria have been developed for diagnosing female urinary obstruction but are not as accurate or as widely accepted because of differences in the physiology of female voiding and the pathology of female urinary obstruction compared with male urinary obstruction. Consequently, videourodynamics during pressure-flow study and consideration of clinical symptoms are typically used to assist in the final diagnosis of female bladder outlet obstruction.

Because of a paucity of literature on detrusor underactivity in both men and women, detrusor underactivity remains a relatively poorly characterized condition without clear objective diagnostic criteria. The modalities used to evaluate detrusor underactivity are the Power (Watt) Factor, the Lin-PURR nomogram, and the BCI Composite

nomogram, all of which were developed to analyze male voiding dysfunction. Overall, further investigation is needed to establish acceptable urodynamic criteria for defining detrusor underactivity in men and women.

REFERENCES

1. Taylor JA, Kuchel GA. Detrusor underactivity: clinical features and pathogenesis of an underdiagnosed geriatric condition. J Am Geriatr Soc 2006;54(12): 1920–32.
2. Griffiths D, Hofner K, van Magstrigt R, et al. Standardization of terminology of lower urinary tract function: pressure-flow studies of voiding, urethral resistance and urethral obstruction. Neurourol Urodyn 1997;16:1–18.
3. Griffiths D. Basics of pressure-flow studies. World J Urol 1995;13:30–3.
4. Nitti VW. Pressure flow urodynamic studies: the gold standard for diagnosing bladder outlet obstruction. Rev Urol 2005;7:S14–21.
5. Nitti VW. Urodynamic and video urodynamic evaluation of lower urinary tract. Campbell Walsh Urology. 10th edition. Philadelphia: Elsevier Health Sciences; 2011.
6. Eri L, Wessel N, Tysland O, et al. Comparative study of pressure-flow parameters. Neurourol Urodyn 2002;21:186–93.
7. Schafer W. Urethral resistance? Urodynamic concepts of physiological and pathological bladder outlet function during voiding. Neurourol Urodyn 1985;4:161–201.
8. Abrams P, Grifith DJ. The assessment of prostatic obstruction from urodynamic measurement and from residual urine. Br J Urol 1979;51:129–34.
9. Lim CS, Abrams P. The Abrams-Griffith nomogram. World J Urol 1995;13:34–9.
10. Abrams PH. Sphincterometry in the diagnosis of male bladder outflow obstruction. J Urol 1976;116: 489–92.

11. Abrams PH. Prostatism and prostatectomy: the value of urine flow rate in the preoperative assessment for operation. J Urol 1977;117:70–1.

12. Abrams PH, Skidmore R, Poole AC, et al. The concept and measurement of bladder work. Br J Urol 1977;49:133–8.

13. Bates CP, Arnold EP, Griffiths DJ. The nature of the abnormality in the bladder neck obstruction. Br J Urol 1975;47:651–6.

14. Griffiths DJ. The mechanics of the urethra and micturition. Br J Urol 1973;45:497–507.

15. Jensen KM, Jorgensen JB, Mogensen P. Urodynamics in prostatism: prognostic value of pressure-flow study combined with stop-flow test. Scand J Urol Nephrol Suppl 1988;144:72–7.

16. Rollema HJ, Magstrigt RV. Improved indication and follow-up in transurethral resection of the prostate using the computer program CLIM: a prospective study. J Urol 1992;148:111–6.

17. Griffiths D, Mastrigt RV, Bosch R. Quantification of urethral resistance and bladder function during voiding, with special reference to the effects of prostate size reduction on urethral obstruction due to benign prostatic hyperplasia. Neurourol Urodyn 1989;8:17–27.

18. Schafer W. Principle and clinical application of advanced urodynamic analysis of voiding function. Urol Clin North Am 1990;17:553–6.

19. Schafer W. The contribution of the bladder outlet to the relation between pressure and flow rate during micturition. In: Hinman F Jr, Boyarsky S, editors. Benign prostatic hypertrophy. New York: Springer-Verlag; 1983. p. 470–96.

20. Blavais J. Multichannel urodynamics studies. Urology 1984;23(5):421–38.

21. Schafer W. Analysis of bladder outlet function with linearized passive urethral resistance relation, linPURR, and disease-specific approach for grading obstruction from complex to simple. World J Urol 1995;13:47–58.

22. Nager CW, Albo M. Testing in women with lower urinary tract dysfunction. Clin Obstet Gynaecol 2004; 47:53–69.

23. Digesu GA, Hutchings A, Salvatore S, et al. Reproducibility and reliability of pressure flow parameters in women. BJOG 2003;110:774–6.

24. Blavais JG, Groutz A. Bladder outlet obstruction nomogram for women with lower urinary tract symptomatology. Neurourol Urodyn 2000;19:553–64.

25. Massey JA, Abrams PH. Obstructed voiding in the female. Br J Urol 1988;61:36–9.

26. Farrar DJ, Osborne JL, Stephenson TP, et al. Urodynamic view of bladder outflow obstruction in the female: factors influencing the results of treatment. Br J Urol 1976;47:815–22.

27. Groutz A, Blavais JG, Chaikin DC. Bladder outlet obstruction in women: definition and characteristics. Neurourol Urodyn 2000;19:213–20.

28. Rees DL, Whitfield HN, Islam AK, et al. Urodynamic findings in females with frequency and dysuria. Br J Urol 1976;47:853–60.

29. Nitti VW, Tu LM, Gitlin J. Diagnosing bladder outlet obstruction in women. J Urol 1999;161:1535–40.

30. Chassagne S, Bernier PA, Haab F, et al. Proposed cutoff value to define bladder outlet obstruction in women. Urology 1998;51:408–11.

31. Lemack GE, Zimmern PE. Pressure flow analysis may aid in identifying women with outflow obstruction. J Urol 2000;163:1823–8.

32. Lemack GE, Basemen AG, Zimmern PE. Voiding dynamics in women: a comparison of pressure-flow studies between asymptomatic and incontinent women. Urology 2002;59:42–6.

33. Defreitas GA, Zimmern PE, Lemack GE, et al. Refining diagnosis of anatomic female bladder outlet obstruction: comparison of pressure flow parameters in clinically obstructed women with those of normal controls. Urology 2004;64:675–9.

34. Cormier L, Ferchaud J, Galas JM, et al. Diagnosis of female outlet obstruction and relevance of the parameter area under the curve of detrussor pressure during voiding: preliminary results. J Urol 2002;167:2083–7.

35. Mahfouz W, Afraa TA, Campeau L, et al. Normal urodynamic parameters in women: part II invasive urodynamics. Int Urogynecol J 2012;23:269–77.

36. Nitti VW, Raz S. Obstruction following anti-incontinence procedures: diagnosis and treatment with transvaginal urethrolysis. J Urol 1994;152(1):93–8.

37. Van Koeveringe GA, Vahabi B, Anderson KE, et al. Detrusor underactivity: a plea for new approaches to common bladder dysfunction. Neurourol Urodyn 2011;30:723–8.

38. Cucchi A, Quaglini S, Rovereto B. Development of idiopathic detrusor underactivity in women: from isolated decrease in contraction velocity to obvious impairment of voiding function. Urology 2008;71(5): 844–8.

39. Cucchi A, Quaglini S, Rovereto B. Proposal for a urodynamic redefinition of detrusor underactivity. J Urol 2009;181:225–9.

40. Cucchi A, Quaglini S, Guarnaschelli C, et al. Urodynamic findings suggestive of two-stage development of idiopathic detrusor underactivity in adult men. Urology 2007;70:75–9.

41. Buttyan R, Chen MW, Levin RM. Animal models of the bladder outlet obstruction and molecular insights into the basis for the development of bladder dysfunction. Eur Urol 1997;32(Suppl 1):32–9.

42. Gosling JA, Kung LS, Dixon JS. Correlation between the structures and function of the rabbit urinary bladder following partial outlet obstruction. J Urol 2000;163:1349–56.

43. Gabella G, Uvelius B. Reversal of muscle hypertrophy in the rat urinary bladder after removal

urethral obstruction. Cell Tissue Res 1994;227: 333–9.

44. Thomas AW, Cannon A, Bartlett E, et al. The natural history of lower urinary tract dysfunction in men: the influence of detrusor underactivity on the outcome after transurethral resection of the prostate with a minimum 10-year urodynamic follow-up. BJU Int 2004;93:745–50.

45. Griffiths DJ, Scholtmeijer RJ. Vesicoureteral reflux and lower urinary tract dysfunction in children: evidence for 2 different reflux/dysfunction complexes. J Urol 1987;137:240–4.

46. Abrams P. Bladder outlet obstruction index, bladder contractility index and bladder voiding efficiency: three simple indices to define bladder voiding function. BJU Int 1999;84:14–5.

Index

Note: Page numbers of article titles are in **boldface** type.

Urol Clin N Am 41 (2014) 469–471
http://dx.doi.org/10.1016/S0094-0143(14)00055-X

urologic.theclinics.com

Moving?

Make sure your subscription moves with you!

To notify us of your new address, find your **Clinics Account Number** (located on your mailing label above your name), and contact customer service at:

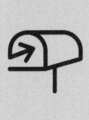

Email: journalscustomerservice-usa@elsevier.com

800-654-2452 (subscribers in the U.S. & Canada)
314-447-8871 (subscribers outside of the U.S. & Canada)

Fax number: 314-447-8029

Elsevier Health Sciences Division
Subscription Customer Service
3251 Riverport Lane
Maryland Heights, MO 63043

ELSEVIER

Printed and bound by CPI Group (UK) Ltd, Croydon, CR0 4YY
03/10/2024
01040376-0010